Health & Fitness for the Road Warrior

Health & Fitness for the Road Warrior

Consistent Fitness by Staying Consistently Healthy

By
Kurt Patrick Gutierrez

Writers Advantage
New York Lincoln Shanghai

Health & Fitness for the Road Warrior
Consistent Fitness by Staying Consistently Healthy

Writers Advantage
an imprint of iUniverse, Inc.

For information address:
iUniverse
2021 Pine Lake Road, Suite 100
Lincoln, NE 68512
www.iuniverse.com

ISBN: 0-595-26079-9

Printed in the United States of America

To Colette, Lauryn and Joseph

Contents

Foreword   vii

Chapter One
You're Off!   1

Chapter Two
Finding Your Personal Why—Your Fitness Mission and Goals   7

Chapter Three
Sleep   13

Chapter Four
Jet Lag   19

Chapter Five
Stress   27

Chapter Six
Eating & Drinking   47

Chapter Seven
Exercise While Traveling   66

Chapter Eight
Returning to the Home Front: Putting It All Together   110

Appendix
Discussion on Heart Rate   113

Foreword

Practical Fitness for the Business Traveler

We have all endured it, suffered through it, and fought like heck to stick to it. No, it's not the *all rice* diet; the proverbial "it" is staying fit while traveling. Traveling on business seems to be especially difficult these days: rich food and drink are in abundance and almost every meeting revolves around a lunch, dinner, or drinks. Though engagements like "business golf" were once a great activity for our health and fitness, we have even found a way to minimize the effort we put into golf. Too often, our exercise consists of getting in and out of the cart to swing a few times and then chase the beer cart.

I wrote this book initially for myself, in an attempt to get healthy. When I traveled on business, invariably I gained weight, got stressed, and didn't sleep well, which weakened my immune system, and I would wind up catching a cold. I was working hard and feeling terrible. I developed the habit of drinking alcohol to help get to sleep and drinking coffee to wake up, which turned into a vicious cycle of unhealthy routines. I wanted to feel good again, to reduce my blood pressure, to maintain my weight, and to stop feeling beat-up and rundown after returning from a few days of business travel. I realized how easy it is to fall into the trap of overindulgence, so I started searching for ways to combat fatigue, bad eating habits, and poor health while traveling on business.

I've always figured that being successful at a health regime was similar to being successful in business. Success in business usually comes from the execution of a well thought-out strategy and thorough planning. Businesspeople understand concepts like budgeting, product development, and the planning process. The types of decisions businesspeople make, the tools they use, and the investments they choose are all crucial in order to be successful in the upcoming fiscal year. Now, take that same approach to planning your next physical health year. Rather than reviewing your expenses and revenues, look at what food and drink you have been ingesting. Just as businesses plan capital expenditures and investments, you should plan a physical fitness regimen and invest in your body and health. Just as we all visualize business success and the wonderful material and esoteric trappings that result from our efforts, so should we visualize a fit, strong, healthy, and lean body.

Staying fit and getting into healthy habits is difficult enough at home; the poor eating habits, stress, lack of sleep, jet lag, and sedentary routine associated with travel make it even harder for today's businessperson to have a healthy lifestyle on the road. The plan described in this book will result in a healthier and potentially more productive life.

Chapter One

You're Off!

Traveling for business can make life seem like a series of hotel rooms, airports and late-night dinners. Your mission is to close the deal, sign the contract, or take care of your customers. Whatever your mission, oftentimes your top priority does not include taking care of yourself. Being healthy and fit while you travel allows you to be more productive, more alert, and more effective. In order to become healthy or to maintain a high fitness level, you should first have a vision of the ideal you. Many people start with great intentions in changing their diets and plan effective exercise programs, only to give up when they encounter obstacles. The key to becoming healthy and fit while traveling is to have a clear sense of your mission, supported by goals and measurable objectives. The program detailed in this book will help you develop personal Health and Fitness goals and ensure you "stick to" your resolutions.

Successful businesspeople understand the processes of goal-setting and using discipline to follow through on strategic/tactical plans. The same process used in setting business and professional goals can and should be used in developing your health and fitness objectives.

Successful businesses have a clear sense of direction and employ many different strategies to attain the vision or mission of a company, which may be to increase shareholder value or to penetrate into new markets. What keeps a business successful is its ability to continue to provide a service or product that customers value. Whatever your business mission, your goals and objectives must be clear, measurable, and attainable. This is not a revolutionary or radical idea. Theodore Levitt, one of the most admired marketers and strategists, states that most businesspeople survive and thrive because their companies have clarified "…[their] purposes, strategies, and plans…[and] that these [are] clearly written down, clearly communicated and frequently reviewed…"[1]

The successful business model requires all of the functional areas of a company to work in conjunction with each other. Operations, Marketing & Sales, Product Development, and Quality are interdependent. If one aspect of the business is not effective or productive, chances are that the entire organization will suffer. When a company has its functional areas operating effectively, the company becomes stronger in the marketplace. If a company continues to have a sustainable competitive advantage, you can expect that company to survive a long time. Similarly, your well-being is dependent upon all aspects of your physical behavior. Your sleep routine, your ability to handle stress, your exercise regime, and your eating and drinking habits all impact overall health: sleeping well helps reduce your stress level; exercising helps you sleep better, relieve stress, and make you more conscientious about your dining habits.

Sleep

Sleeping well helps to keep us healthy, rejuvenating our bodies and repairing our immune systems. Business travel causes us to change time zones, sleep in strange places, and stress over important meetings, all of which contribute to the disruption of a normal night's sleep. The average person needs six to eight hours of uninterrupted (and non-drug induced) sleep in order to feel refreshed. Lack of sleep can make us

---

[1] Theodore Levitt, *The Marketing Imagination*, (New York, N.Y.: The Free Press, 1986), 6.

more susceptible to colds, cause grogginess, and may lead to poor job performance.

If you are sleeping well at home, you can develop techniques to help you more easily enter slumberland on the road. While you are traveling, you can apply the same routines or nightly rituals that prepare you for bed at home. You should also examine those common obstacles to sleep like caffeine, late heavy dinners, worry, stress, and physical discomfort. If you reduce or eliminate those sleep obstacles and keep a routine, sleeping should be a stress-free and refreshing endeavor.

Jet Lag

Jet lag typically occurs when the traveler crosses into new time zones. Changing your meal schedule to coincide with that of your destination's schedule will significantly help to reduce jet lag. The phenomena of travel and jet lag can have lots of negative side effects, specifically: fatigue, dehydration, and disruption in your sleep patterns. Astronauts, pilots, and political leaders have found ways to cope with jet lag. Business travelers can use the same types of techniques to reduce or eliminate the effects of jet lag.

Stress

Business travel is stressful. Oftentimes, the most stressful aspects of our travel are those that are beyond our direct control. Sometimes the plane is late, or there are traffic delays, crowds of people, and various incidents that slow us down against our will. Life on the road is full of unexpected events: stressors invade our lives always at the wrong time and place. While we cannot necessarily control what happens to us, we *can* control how we respond to stressful situations. Internalizing stress can have devastating effects on our lives, often causing health issues that range from depression to anxiety to heart disease.

Not all stress, however, is bad stress. Sometimes these events that "stress" us also provide excitement to our lives, a reason to respond, a reason to get out of bed in the morning. The same event or issue that can make one person sick with worry can make another giddy with excitement. The difference is in the attitude (mindset) of the individual. With the correct attitude and preparation we can choose how we react to those unpredictable events. We can choose to find the positive in all situations, and maybe even some humor. If there is a certain event or unavoidable stressor that really angers or hurts us, we still can find a way to relieve that stress. If you feel like the weight of the world is on your shoulders, simply breathing, practicing some stress relief techniques, exercising, and finding some humor in the situation will reduce the tension and some of your misery.

Exercise

Exercise programs, home exercise equipment, and health spas are all very popular today. In some cases, your hotel may have available facilities or may even give you a free pass to a nearby gym. However, many business travelers use the inconvenience of their trip as an ostensible reason for not exercising. The most common excuses are associated with a lack of time and a lack of energy. Many travelers view exercise as pure drudgery. If, however, you have sincerely developed your mission with measurable objectives, your excuses will be eliminated. Your mission will give you the "fire in the belly" necessary to integrate exercise into your overall health effort.

Contrary to popular opinion, exercise does not have to be boring. There are plenty of ways to enjoy your exercises. Taking a power walk through an interesting part of town or a nice park is a great form of exercise and stress relief. Playing a pick-up basketball game, playing a couple of rounds of golf, or going for a run helps loosen up those muscles after a long day's travel. In this book, we have incorporated exercise routines for business travelers who are just beginning an exercise program, for those who are already in good shape, and also for those committed few who are in excellent shape.

Eating

Regardless of your exercise program, you still need to eat right. If that age-old adage "you are what you eat" were correct, many of our contemporaries would be jelly donuts. Business travelers are forever tempted to eat more food and drink more alcohol. Most social business meetings and events revolve around meals and cocktails. We all love to partake of those rich meals; moderation, however, is the key to maintaining both your waistline and your health.

Returning Home

Your return home can also be quite unsettling. Many business travelers expect the world to come to a screeching halt until they return. We are secretly disappointed when our family and friends have gone on living their lives without us. The traveler can find ways to ease the transition back home and back to work. The most important aspect of a happy return is in steady communication and planning. Your spouse, family, and friends will appreciate your efforts to continue to be part of their lives even when you're not physically present. Calling, sending a postcard, or firing off a quick e-mail helps let your loved ones know you care. At work, communicating with both your superiors and your direct reports is essential for conducting your business. Being out of the "communication loop" can have a devastating effect on your career as well your ability to add value immediately upon your return to the workplace. If you have been keeping up with e-mail and voicemail while traveling, you are less likely to be overwhelmed by these items when you are back in action.

Being healthy and fit will help every aspect of your life. You will feel better, look better, and probably be more effective at your job. To be inspired to get and stay fit, find out what motivates you, then plan your strategy and take action.

Chapter Two

Finding Your Personal Why—Your Fitness Mission and Goals

The corporate visioning process = personal commitment

> In the long run, men only hit what they aim at.
> —Henry David Thoreau

A clear set of goals, a plan, a sincere desire, and definitive action to attain your objectives will almost always ensure success. Your aims for health and fitness at home should be the same as they are while you are traveling. What you learn in this book will help you start the process immediately, whether you picked this book up at the airport bookstore or ordered it via the Internet and had it delivered to your home. Being healthy and fit will positively affect all aspects of your life. When you make an effort to get rid of those "love handles" by eating better and working out, you'll find that you are able to sleep more soundly, concentrate better, and relieve stress. This book takes the holistic approach to health and fitness: exercise programs, stress relief techniques, and healthy eating suggestions all work together to provide a complete plan to achieve optimal health.

Travel throws even health-conscious people a curve ball. Business traveling can lead to overeating, sleep deprivation, and jet lag, all of which take a toll on your immune system. Many business travelers choose to reward themselves for the hours spent away from home by eating exotic foods and drinking more alcoholic beverages than they would normally consume. Indulging in the additional nightcap or extra dessert is especially difficult on your body while traveling, since your tight schedule often keeps you going from early morning to late evening. The stress of being away from loved ones, participating in important meetings, and changing time zones can decrease your productivity, effectiveness, and wreck havoc on your overall health. If it seems like you can't find the time to take care of yourself while traveling, think of the alternative: a tired, sick, fat, and sluggish you. You *can* fit in your health regimen. In fact, when you feel better, you work more efficiently and perform better professionally.

Getting fit, sleeping better, relieving stress, and losing weight may sound like difficult goals to achieve. If you are a stressed out, overweight road warrior, your fitness goals will be more accessible if you tie those objectives to your mission, then break them down into a series of smaller goals, each having a high probability of success. Your fitness mission should be a statement of your personal philosophy about health and its effect on the quality of your life. What are your reasons for wanting to accomplish a certain health and fitness goal? For example, you might want to lose weight and be more alert during meetings on the road. Maybe you want to train for that marathon while on the road and finish with a competitive time, or maybe you just want to lose that extra 15 pounds you've been carrying around your waist. Maybe you would just like to recognize the person in the mirror who grew that triple chin.

Writing a mission statement may seem like a daunting task, considering many companies hire "strategist consultants" to help them along. We can simplify the process by providing a step-by-step guide for developing your personal mission. Writing down your mission statement will help you understand what your goals are and how you will measure those goals. Your mission, clearly stated, will help you fulfill the vision you have of yourself. The following exercise will help identify the personal fitness and health mission specific to your needs.

Exercise: Health and Fitness Mission Statement Development

Time: 15 minutes
Equipment: paper & pencil
Instructions: Write down a list of your personal reasons for staying fit and healthy. Here are a few thoughts to help you start your exercise: Why do you value being healthy? What physical/psychological feelings do you want to experience while traveling? How will being health conscious and following through on your exercise program make you feel about yourself? How will it affect the things you care about? Will you derive satisfaction from being in touch with your physical self? What motivates you to do any exercise or take care of your body, at home or away? Is there a sport you will be better at, a special someone to look better for, or are you simply tired of constantly feeling fatigued while traveling? Are you seeking more enjoyment and a higher quality of life? Are you invested in building your immune system or working on disease prevention? Answering these questions should lead you to discover your personal fitness/health mission statement. Next, consolidate your ideas into a concise statement. Following are some examples of mission statements.

Examples of a Fitness/Health Mission Statement:

1. I want to feel good about the way I treat my body. I realize I only have one body and I must nurture it and keep it free of sickness and pain. I am investing in my health because I value my life and I want my children to follow my example and respect their bodies.
2. I value freedom most of all. One of the keys to a high-quality life is freedom from chronic fatigue, illness, and pain. I will do all that I

can to rid myself of those unhealthy habits that will reduce my quality of life.

Goals and Objectives

Establishing a clear vision and mission of your healthy self will help you in defining your personal goals. Your goals are what you want to accomplish to support your mission. Your objectives are the specific measurements that support your larger goals. *Remember:* all things are created twice; once in the mind, and then in reality. Just as the architect visualizes and designs a home before it's built, you should visualize the new healthy and fit you. To speed up the goal-setting process, I have broken down the list of typical problem areas experienced while traveling. Use the following goal setting-guidelines; please make these goals very personal and adjust accordingly.

1. **Set specific and measurable objectives with timetables.** If your goal is to lose weight, your objective should say *how much* you want to lose and by *when.*

2. **Choose difficult but realistic goals.** If your goals are unrealistic, you may become discouraged even though you have made progress. However, don't set your goals too low. As they say in the United States Army, strive to "be all that you can be."

3. **Take small steps in achieving your goals.** Say "I will lose one pound every two weeks," rather than "I will lose 30 pounds this month."

4. **Write down mission, goals, and objectives.** I have provided a template to list your goals and objectives. If you write down your goals and refer to them often, you have a much higher chance of achieving them and carrying out your mission.

5. **Develop a goal achievement plan.** Write down *how* you are going to achieve your goals. The strong plan of attack will provide a road map and guide you to attaining your objectives.

6. **Develop good habits.** Once is not enough; you have to work conscientiously over a sustained period until your healthy practices become habits.

7. **Develop goal support.** Let others know what your fitness goals are. Most people will support you. Letting your family know what your goals are can be especially helpful.

8. **Develop evaluation.** Your progress toward your goal may not always be steady. You'll need continuous feedback and evaluation of how you're doing. Keep a close eye on your progress: get on the scale often, measure your distance or newest run time.

Exercise: Travel Health Issues and Proposed Goals

Time: 15 min
Equipment: pencil and paper
Instructions: Write out your goals, or what you want to accomplish, in bullet points or in long form. Use whatever method feels more comfortable for you. Your objectives will measure your success. The achievement plan will provide the "how" for accomplishing your goals and objectives. The following is an example of a goals, objects, and achievement plan:

<u>Issue</u>	<u>Example Goals/Objectives/Achievement Plan</u>
Diet	Eat better on the road
	Lose 5 lbs. per month
	Reduce junk food consumption
Sleep	Be well-rested while traveling
	Sleep soundly for seven consecutive hours
	Remove sleep obstacles

Exercise	Stay in shape even when schedules are constrained
	Reduce resting heart rate to 68 beats per minute
	Start walking program
Stress	Reduce travel/business related stress
	Reduce blood pressure/headaches
	Learn stress relief techniques
Jet Lag	Feel fit after long flights
	Overcome jet lag
	Use specific jet lag techniques

Now it's your turn. Write out your personal goals in the chart provided.

Issue	Goals/Objectives/Achievement Plan
Diet	_____
Sleep	_____
Jet Lag	_____
Exercise	_____
Stress	_____

Congratulations. Once you have completed your personalized mission, goals, and objectives, you have completed the most difficult aspect of your road to health and fitness. By writing and personalizing these goals, you have greatly increased the likelihood that you will achieve your desired outcome. If your mission statement is based upon what you really value, you can make fitness while traveling a habit. You can plan your day-to-day health regimen as well and make it an extension of your overall goals.

The remainder of this book will give you ideas, techniques, and plans, and will help propel you forward to achieving your goals. If you follow the guidelines and make the effort, I will guarantee your success or refund the money spent on this book.

Chapter Three

Sleep

Business Applications:

Investing in critical resources and resource recovery = sleeping soundly

> The best cure for insomnia is to get a lot of sleep.
> —W. C. Fields

> No small art is it to sleep: it is necessary for that purpose to keep awake all day.
> —Friedrich W. Nietzsche[2]

It's four o'clock in the morning. You glance at the hotel clock. It angrily stares back at you. You've been wrestling with your pillows all night and the pillows are winning. You start to panic. Tomorrow you have a very important business meeting and you need to be at your best. You are frustrated, anxious, angry, and exhausted, yet you can't get to sleep.

Does this story sound familiar?

If your sleep is affected by traveling, it will impact your overall well-being. We all need sleep to heal us, to repair our immune system, and to help fight off stress. Here are some important tips on sleep:

---

[2] http://www.landandsky.com/quotes.html

- It is more important to have some continuous sleep than a lot of fragmented sleep.

- There is no "normal" amount of sleep. The amount of sleep time each individual requires varies dramatically from person to person.

- Travel, stress, and exercise increase the need for rest and can affect your sleep patterns.

- The key is to know how much sleep you need. You can gauge this by remembering a time when you woke feeling rested and weren't tired again until bedtime.

- Travelers' insomnia is caused when your biological clock becomes confused, for example, when you change time zones. I will cover jet lag in chapter four.

Initially, we will discuss the obstacles that prevent you from getting a good night's sleep. Eliminating these "sleep obstacles" will dramatically improve your chances of sleeping restfully through the night. The second part of this chapter discusses ways to change your mental and physical environment so you can increase the likeliness of getting a good night's sleep. Select a few of these methods and incorporate them into your goals.

Sleep Obstacles: All the Things That Keep You from Entering LaLa Land

- **Exercising too close to bedtime.** Exercising *is* important in helping you sleep. However, if you exercise fewer than three hours before sleeping, you will "wake" the body by increasing your metabolic rate. You will then be too "revved up" to settle down.

- **Caffeine.** Drink coffee, tea, or cola no closer than five hours before bedtime, or you will be counting the tiles on the ceiling. Drink decaffeinated coffee after dinner (unless you are one of those few who are immune to the effects of caffeine).

- **Late Dinners.** Sometimes late dinners are unavoidable. If your business involves a late dinner, try to eat on the lighter side. Heavy dinners may cause trouble digesting and keep you awake at night. A better habit is to eat a big breakfast or lunch and a lighter dinner. Do not, however, try a starvation diet while traveling. Eating too little may keep you awake at night—hungry and rummaging for change for the vending machine holding that precious Snickers bar.

- **Smoking.** Skip the after-dinner cigar or cigarette. Nicotine is a stimulant and can disrupt sleep.

- **Dehydration.** Traveling, especially by air, will dehydrate your body. The pressurized atmosphere in planes has notoriously "bad" recycled air. It may wreak havoc on your sinuses and keep you up at night with a stuffy nose. Try to drink at least eight glasses of water a day. You can't drink too much water (unless it's too close to bedtime, in which case you'll be up all night voiding your system).

- **Alcohol.** Go ahead and have one or two drinks if that's part of your normal routine. Be careful: drinking alcohol on a flight seems to intensify its effect. A glass of wine is supposed to good for your health, but don't overdo it. That extra nightcap will help you drift off to sleep, but may result in lighter, more fragmented sleep.

- **Watching the local news.** The local news increases its ratings by showing all the *bad* news. I can't figure it out, but people love to turn it on and watch how many people were shot or stabbed in their lovely city. The local reports tend to be filled with a lot of violent stories and just really bad news. The mayhem on the streets may cause you to worry excessively about your loved ones at home. Stick to the business news—it has everything you need to know anyway.

Just as there are many obstacles to your sleep, there are many factors that can *help* you rest as well. The following list of physical and mental factors can be changed or controlled to suit your needs:

- **Exercise early in the day.** Your body will be refreshed during most of the day and naturally start to wind down during the evening. This strategy works especially efficiently if you can exercise before you get on an airplane.

- **Read.** Pick up a good book (or a bad book!) until your eyes get heavy.

- **Keep you hotel room comfortably cool**—65 degrees Fahrenheit works for most people. Most people sleep better warm and snug under the covers in a cooler room.

- **Turn the hotel clock radio away from you** so you don't wake up and stare at it all night.

- Try to **reduce the noise** in and around your hotel room. Request a room some distance from elevators and stairways. Also, make sure your room is not facing a busy street. Try using earplugs and eye patches to eliminate excess noise and light, allowing you to sleep more soundly.

- **Hunger.** If you are hungry, eat some bananas or drink some low-fat milk. You may have to plan for this ahead of time by swiping the bananas, milk, or cereal that morning from the continental breakfast, or stopping by a local grocery store.

- **Dress comfortably.** If you wear pajamas at home, wear them at the hotel. If you usually sleep in your birthday suit, do the same at the hotel. (Be sure to double-check the cleanliness of the sheets, though.)

The key to restful sleep while traveling is to maintain a routine on the road that is as similar as possible to what you do when you are at home (and presumably sleeping well). Planning will always be the key to successful, healthy travel. If you find that you still have trouble falling asleep, do not force yourself. In fact, you can't force yourself to sleep. Get out of bed and stretch or try the following relaxation technique.

Sleep/Relaxation Techniques

Later we will address stress relief and meditation. The following exercise works well to relieve both stress and insomnia. I've found that this exercise works best for me in trying to get to sleep when I'm stressed.

Lie flat on your back, arms comfortable at your side, legs straight. Breathe in deeply through your nose and exhale through your mouth. Inhale deeply, hold your breath, make a fist with your right hand and squeeze as hard as you can. Strain the entire right arm while your face and the rest of your body is relaxed and remains still. Hold your breath and the tension, squeezing hard for 10 seconds. Slowly exhale. As you exhale, release the tension from your arm and say to yourself "relax" or whatever word helps you calm yourself. Imagine your arm being heavy and feel the tension from your arm falling away. Repeat the process on each arm twice, then repeat the process on your legs. After your arms and legs are totally relaxed, continue to breathe calmly and say to yourself "relaxed and heavy." Even if this exercise doesn't put you to sleep immediately, it will help alleviate the tension behind your insomnia.

Habits and Sleep

As I mentioned earlier, we tend to drift off to sleep more quickly if we have a set routine. While it is difficult to have routine and structure while traveling, any routine is still better than not having one at all. Here is a routine that works well for almost anyone and it takes 30 to 50 minutes. Don't get stressed if you don't do all of these things:

- Call your loved ones and say good night.
- Brush and floss your teeth.

- Take a warm bath.
- Do some light stretching exercises.
- Do your relaxation techniques or mediation.
- Say your prayers.

Chapter Four

Jet Lag

It's four o'clock in the afternoon and you're feeling groggy during a session of very important business negotiations. You flew into town the day before, traveling through two time zones. You wish you had toothpicks to keep your eyes from closing; you feel mentally fuzzy and slow. You have to be at your best, but you know you're stumbling your way through this meeting. You've probably got jet lag.

In this global community, businesspeople travel across countries and continents to interface directly with their customers and vendors. While the Internet, wireless communications, and other technological advances have made our business dealings more efficient, face-to-face interaction is still vital to our success. Therefore, business travel is a necessity. For me, the glamour of globetrotting lasted about three minutes; it was even less for some of my colleagues. Business schools don't tell us how to overcome the traveling consequences of feeling drained, fatigued, and dehydrated. Jet lag is basically a disruption of the biological clock that affects everyone to varying degrees. First, we'll identify the symptoms and then we will discuss some techniques for overcoming jet lag.

Jet Lag Symptoms

Fatigue

Jet lag can leave you feeling fatigued, worn out, and tired for days after your arrival. It is usually accompanied by the inability to concentrate.

Disorientation

Have you ever lost your hotel or car rental key, only to find it in your luggage after you return home? Forgetfulness and what seems like early signs of Alzheimer's disease are symptomatic of jet lag. This phenomenon is especially embarrassing when you're with customers.

Fragmented Sleep

Do you find that you're dying to sleep during the day and can't get to sleep at night? NASA estimates that travelers need one day for every time zone they cross in order to regain their normal rhythm and energy levels. That means that for a five-hour time difference, you'll require five days to get back to peak performance. I do not know of any business traveler who has the luxury of *one* day, let alone five.

Being confined for hours on end only serves to aggravate the symptoms of jet lag. Here are some physical issues to deal with while you're on the plane:

Dehydration

The pressurized air in the cabin of a commercial airplane is very dry. This can cause headaches, dry skin, nasal irritation, and make you more susceptible to any colds, coughs, sore throats, and flu that are always floating around in the aircraft. After all, you're sharing that recycled air.

Discomfort in legs and feet

When you get dehydrated, your feet, ankles, hands, and limbs swell, especially during an extended flight. This can be extremely uncomfortable. There have been times, due to swelling, that my feet felt as though they were being strangled by the spandex in my socks, and I have been unable to comfortably put my shoes back on.

Preventing (Or at Least Minimizing) Jet Lag

Your Pre-Flight Condition

As we discussed earlier, try to be well-rested before you begin your trip. If you're overly-tired, excited, stressed, nervous, or hung-over before the flight, you are probably going to feel the effects of jet lag. If you are very sick with a cold and fever, try to delay your trip until you're feeling better.

Hydrate Yourself

Drinking lots of water helps. Take a bottle of water with you! Some airlines supply water frequently to passengers, but others only have a small water fountain near the toilets. Coffee, tea, alcoholic drinks, and sodas are diuretics and will cause your body to expel fluid. Water is the magical liquid that can keep you well, and your body craves it.

Alcohol

The open bar atmosphere in business class provides an opportunity to overindulge, but remember that the impact of alcohol on the body is two to three times more potent when you're flying. That means that one glass of wine in-flight has the effect of two to three glasses on the ground. Add this to the other problems listed above, and you can get off the plane with a huge hangover that simply compounds the already detrimental effects of jet lag.

Food and drink

Airline coffee and tea seem to have higher then usual caffeine content. If you don't drink a lot of coffee or can do without it, then do without. You don't need them—especially when flying. Also, beware of potentially risky foods served on some airlines in certain parts of the world, including salads, cold meat, and fish.

Lack of exercise

Lack of exercise is one of the worst aspects of long-haul flying. It makes the flight even more uncomfortable and sets you up for a longer period of jet lag afterwards. Do the exercises I have outlined later in this chapter. Try to get up every 30 to 45 minutes and walk the aisles. Get your blood moving—don't just allow it to pool up in your ankles.

Wash up

If you get an extended layover, look for facilities to take a shower. If no facility exists, then wash your face and brush your teeth. Doing even a small amount of personal grooming will refresh you (and make you more tolerable to your fellow passengers).

Techniques for Reducing the Effects of Jet Lag

Sleeping aids

Sleeping on the plane, if you can, will help you arrive refreshed. Blindfolds, ear plugs, neck rests and blow-up neck pillows are all useful in helping you get quality sleep while flying. Kick your shoes off to ease the pressure on the feet and bring some comfortable socks to wear. Some airlines provide soft, sock-like slippers, and many seasoned travelers carry their own.

Melatonin (See http://www.melatonin.com)

Noted author of *PilotVision* and personal friend, John Magness, flew helicopters with the military's special operations helicopter group called the Night Stalkers. Most of the Night Stalkers' operations were at night, leaving John open to the effects of jet lag. Consequently, he swears by melatonin. Melatonin is a natural hormone produced by the pineal gland which sets the body's schedule of sleeping and waking—its circadian rhythm. Cued by nightfall, melatonin production increases tenfold, triggering many of the physiological changes that accompany sleep. In the right doses, it makes you feel like you're ready to go to bed. And, unlike sleeping pills, melatonin allows you to wake up feeling refreshed.

Studies indicate that after taking a melatonin supplement, a person may reset his or her body clock to nighttime, regardless of the time of day. International travelers may be able to decrease the effects of jet lag by taking melatonin at strategic times over a period of days, thus setting the body clock to a new time zone.

Is melatonin the wonder drug? According to Mayo Clinic specialists, the answer is no, for several reasons. First, caution is warranted because the long-term effects of melatonin supplements are unknown. Also, melatonin is currently sold as a food supplement, so its manufacture and marketing are not subject to the strict pharmaceutical standards of the Food and Drug Administration. Furthermore, as a treatment for the effects of jet lag, melatonin is both controversial and complex; the latest research shows that if used incorrectly, melatonin will make jet lag worse! Can't sleep? Talk to your doctor! At this point, melatonin may have promise. But the final verdict is not in.

Sleeping Pills

Don't do it. Many travelers use sleeping pills to try to alleviate jet lag, sometimes with disastrous results. In 1988, the *Lancet* estimated that, "over three years at Heathrow Airport, 18% of the 61 sudden deaths in long distance passengers were caused by clots in the lungs."[3] One of the most dangerous aspects of sleeping pills is that they induce a comatose state that allows little or no natural body movement. Imagine your legs'

---

[3] http://jetlag.co.nz

veins as bags of blood and muscle. When this blood doesn't circulate, there is an increased possibility that it will clot. Another trouble with sleeping pills: many are variants on antihistamines and tend to exacerbate the already problematic condition of dehydration.

Anti-Jet Lag Diet

Another method is the Argonne Anti-Lag Diet. This diet is for people who have a lot of time and patience. Though it's relatively complicated, many travelers swear by it:

The Argonne National Laboratory Anti-Jet-Lag Diet[4]
The Argonne Anti-Jet-Lag Diet helps travelers quickly adjust their bodies' internal clocks to new time zones. It is also being used to speed the adjustment of shiftworkers, such as powerplant operators, to periodically rotating work hours. The diet was developed by Dr. Charles F. Ehret of Argonne's Division of Biological and Medical Research as an application of his fundamental studies of the daily biological rhythms of animals. Argonne National Laboratory is one of the US Department of Energy's major centers for research in energy and the fundamental sciences. I have tried this once and it has worked extremely well for me. The process, however, is cumbersome and requires a good deal of planning and foresight. Therefore it may not be effective for you "pull it off in the last minute" artists. See http://jetlag.co.nz/.

How to Avoid Jet Lag[5]

1.   Determine the breakfast time at destination of day of arrival.

---

[4] http://www.slip.net/~mschnapp/jetlag.html.
[5] Argonne National Laboratory, 9700 South Cass Avenue, Argonne, Illinois 60439
   *U.S. Government printing office 1984-754-904

2. Follow the diet schedule *feast/fast/ feast/fast* on *home time.* Start three days before departure day.

Use home time for the following:

Day 1	<u>Feast</u>
Day 2	<u>Fast</u>
Day 3	<u>Feast</u>
Day 4	<u>Fast</u>
Departure Day	<u>Going west?</u> Fast only half day.

Notes to coffee and Coke fiends:

<u>Going east?</u>: Only between 6 and 11 p.m.

<u>Going west?</u>: Take them in the morning.

Use Destination Time:

Sleep	But rise at breakfast time
Breakfast	• Wake up and **Feast**
	• Have a high-protein breakfast.
	• Lights on.
	• Stay awake and active.
Remaining meals	Follow your normal meal schedule.

No alcohol on the plane.

No alcohol on the plane.

Feast

- Breakfast   High-protein meals to stimulate the body's active cycle.
- Lunch   Suitable meals include:
    - steak,
    - eggs,
    - hamburgers,
    - high-protein cereals, and
    - green beans.

- Dinner   High-carbohydrate meal to stimulate sleep.
                They include:
    - spaghetti and other pastas (but no meatballs),
    - crepes (but no meat filling),
    - potatoes,
    - other starchy vegetables, and
    - sweet desserts.

Fast

FAST days help deplete the liver's store of carbohydrates and prepare the body's clock for resetting.
Suitable foods include:

- fruit,
- light soups,
- broths,
- skimpy salads,
- unbuttered toast, and
- half pieces of bread.

    Keep calories and carbohydrates to a minimum.

Chapter Five

Stress

Most people are abo ut as happy as they make up their minds to be.
—Abraham Lincoln[6]

It's not stress that kills us, it is our reaction to it.
—Hans Selye

Worry never robs tomorrow of its sorrow, it only saps today of its joy.
—Leo Buscaglia[7]

You're rushing to pack your bags, your flight leaves in two hours, and you are 45 minutes from the airport (with no traffic). You still need to pick up your presentation and business cards from work, which is 15 minutes' drive in the wrong direction. You're starting to sweat! Eventually you make it to the airport and find your way through the check-in line. You make it to your seat, sweating, stressed, and disheveled, only to realize that you forgot your business cards.

Traveling causes stress. Something unexpected is bound to come up. Even though there is no avoiding stress, you can develop skills for reducing its effects. The keys to managing stress are planning, preparation,

---

[6] http://www.aphids.com/cgi-bin/quotes.pl?act=ShowListingsForCat&Category=L
[7] http://www.aphids.com/cgi-bin/quotes.pl?act=ShowListingsForSub&Subject=S18

and using techniques for relief. My brother-in-law once told me, "If you're stressed out over something, write your feelings on paper and then throw that piece of paper away. That way, you throw your stress out too." My brother-in-law's common sense approach to stress relief has recently been shown to have some validity. A study in the *Journal of the American Medical Association* reported that writing down your stressful thoughts might help provide relief from such illness.[8] Stress is your reaction to stressors—those conditions or events that cause stress. Stressors can be internal (feeling frustrated or having a negative outlook) or external (missing your airplane flight, getting stuck in traffic, or making a presentation in front of a hostile audience).

Stress impacts our immune systems. When we are stressed, our bodies are in the "fight or flight" mode, like animals trying to save their lives. Just like what happens to zebras as they try to escape lions on the African plains, adrenaline pumps through our system, our heart rate increases, and our muscles tense as we run away from the proverbial stress lion.

When something causes us stress, our brain decides to either fight or flee, and then signals the body to build for strength, speed, and power. The adrenal glands begin an immediate outpouring of adrenaline, which raises our heart rate, increases our respiration, and redirects blood flow to our limbs; the mouth gets dry, and the stomach stops digesting. The adrenaline rush into our bloodstream is meant to save our lives in a dangerous situation. The problem, however, is that our bodies cannot handle the continual flood of adrenaline into our bloodstream. Research has shown that stress can cause chronic fatigue (you're constantly running from that lion), depression, high blood pressure,

---

[8] David Speigel, "Healing Words-Emotional Expression and Disease Outcome." *MD.* (April 14, 1999): page#.

viral infections (because your immune system is weakened), and all sorts of life-shortening illnesses. For more information, visit: http://www.4stress.com/main.shtml.

Identifying Stressors

Where is the stress coming from when you travel? Take an inventory of those areas in your life that stress you. You might be able to eliminate more than you realize.

Relationships

Relationships of any kind can be a source of either stress or a stress-release. Often they're both. Is the guy/gal you're traveling with a jerk, or does it help to have someone to work/travel with? If it's difficult traveling with someone, figure out a way to meet him/her at the airport and do not sit together.

Work

If you're not currently in a job or career that's fulfilling or engaging, do your best to make it more satisfying. Throw yourself into your work as if it were your passion. Be positive and your work will be more rewarding. If it sounds a little too simple, try it anyway. No one but you controls your attitude.

Lack of Sleep

Our bodies need sleep. As stated earlier, sleep heals our bodies and gives us coping mechanisms to help deal with life's little crises.

Not Enough Exercise

Exercise releases endorphins into the bloodstream and makes you feel good. Exercise will get your mind off what troubles you, thus preventing and relieving stress.

Worry

In his book, *Don't Sweat the Small Stuff…and It's All Small Stuff*, Dr. Richard Carlson uses the "100 year rule." Meaning, ask yourself this question: in 100 years will what I am presently worrying about be important? Think about the last five years. Better yet, think about last year. Can you remember what you were worried about on a particular day last year? Worrying is just a habit. It is something we can choose to control. The "100 year rule" is one of many methods that help to break this painful and destructive habit.[9]

Personal Safety and Security

The terrorist attacks on September 11, 2001 have changed the travelers' world and our sense of security forever. We no longer feel safe walking down the streets of our Nation's capital or in our great financial centers. We Roadwarriors have to wait in seemingly endless lines and have strangers dig through our personal belongings. The heightened security, while necessary, adds frustration and expends precious time.

International travel adds other significant challenges. All travelers are targets for crime. Criminals seek us travelers out because we appear to be easy prey. Intenational Roadwarriors are always familiar with their immediate surroundings. As we stray into strange waters these criminals

---

[9] Paraphrased from Richard Carlson's audio tape *DON'T SWEAT THE SMALL STUFF…and It's All Small Stuff*, an Abridgement of *Don't Sweat the Small Stuff and It's all Small Stuff* (New York, NY: Simon and Schuster, 1997).

act like sharks and try to pick us off. I have had a few incidents in shark infested waters myself. The first was in the "safest country in the world"…Sweden. My colleagues and I had a lunch appointment with a major customer. We all went to into our customer's facility to briefly introduce ourselves and then we were to provide transportation to the restaurant. Our vehicle was locked and parked inside a gated and moni-tored business compound. The local Sales Representative said, "We'll be back in a few minutes, leave your stuff here…it will be fine". Upon our return, only 10 minutes later, the vehicle was opened with a "slim Jim" (professional thief's trade mark tool) and all our possessions were gone. Passports, luggage, clothes and even our sales samples and collaterals were taken. What a hassle! We did not close the deal even though our customer felt sorry for us. There are no totally secure compounds. Trust nothing to security guards with whom you are not familiar. Be wary of an overly friendly stranger asking you for directions as their partner tries to steal your computer or your briefcase. Do not advertise that you are unfamiliar to the area. This serves as a beacon for would be bad guys.

In a separate incident, I remember arriving in Bangkok, Thailand at 1:00 am for the first time after an 8-hour flight from Australia. What Chaos! As I walked through security no less then 5 people were grab-bing at my luggage pulling me in 5 different directions. I felt accosted and confused and angry. My adrenaline was at its maximum and my body was debating Fight them all or Flight from the scene. It took me a while to realize these people were taxi cab drivers and were vying for my business. Once in the cab, I had no idea if the cab driver was taking me to the correct hotel or to some dark alley where his partners lay in wait to rob me or worse. I got to the hotel safe and sound, but extremely frazzled. I could have saved myself a tremendous amount of unneces-sary stress and headache if I had prepared better.

American travelers are the targets of terrorists. If you are traveling abroad, do your homework and research the place you will visit. My brother, Karl, has been with the State Department for over 20 years. He has been responsible for the personal security for Secretary of States: Colin Powell, Madeline Albreit, and George Schultz as well as countless political dignitaries. He has traveled extensively and worked in security for US Embassies in London and Paris. He has seen attacks on US personnel in the Middle East and across the world.

Karl tells us one of the simplest ways to avoid travel stress is to have your agent or country representative familiar with the territory meet you and pre-arrange all the travel and hotels. It may seem like common sense but sometimes we tend to be over confident about the "little things". My brother also recommends doing homework on cities or countries were you are about to visit. He has provided some great web sites that will give updates on the local tensions, political unrest, and places to avoid. Sites to visit before your visit/trip: www.ds-osac.org (Overseas Security Advisory Council), www.fema.gov (Federal Emergency Management Agency), www.state.gov, www.travel.state.gov, www.hazmat.dot.gov (US Dept of transportation), and www.tsa.dot.gov/public/index.jsp (Transportation Security Agency).

Skills for Managing Stress

Planning and Preparation

In the military and in the business world, there is a pithy phrase that's used often: "Piss poor planning leads to piss poor performance." The same is true of business travelers: trip planning and preparation will minimize the number of issues we will face. Prepare for your trip at least two days before you depart. Plan for unexpected emergency trips as well by keeping an overnight bag packed in your closet. When you pack, make sure you have what you need from the office ready to go. Your computer, trade magazines you plan to read, and whatever else you'll need to bring with you should be part of your packing effort. If you wait to "finish" your packing at the office, you will more than likely find yourself out of space in your luggage or briefcase. Last-minute running around will cause unnecessary stress and will probably cause you to forget something important.

Mentally plan out your agenda. Write it down and give it to your loved one at home. This will help you prepare and pack properly and let your children, spouse, or significant other know where you are and what you are doing. Items to include are: flight times, hotel telephone numbers, and reservation confirmation numbers. Here is a checklist to help you pack:

Professional Material

- ❑ Laptop
- ❑ Computer associated software, floppy, CD, battery recharger, electrical adapters, phone cables.
- ❑ Presentation materials
- ❑ Cell phone, battery recharger
- ❑ Documents.
- ❑ Business cards
- ❑ Professional magazines and reading material
- ❑ Writing material and instruments
- ❑ Phone numbers & Internet access numbers (AT&T Worldnet will send you a diskette of local access numbers by calling (1-888-428-8527), or you can download them from: http://www.worldnet.att.

(Always carry your professional material with you as you board the plane. Lost articles have ruined too many careers.)

Travel

- ❑ Tickets. I don't like e-ticket for International travel. Regular airplane tickets are like possessing currency. It's much easier to negotiate when you have an actual ticket in your hand. In the US e-tickets counters are readily available and relatively simple to access.
- ❑ Reservation numbers: rental car, hotel, flight
- ❑ Credit cards, cash, travelers' checks
- ❑ Identification documents—Make one copy of your passport in case of theft.
- ❑ Itinerary. Make an extra copy to leave with your family.

Personal

- ❑ Photos of loved ones
- ❑ Leave your name and address in your bags, just in case of loss
- ❑ Pack your toiletry and essentials in a <u>clear</u> plastic bag so the security agent can see what you have and will not have to open your kit.
- ❑ Bottled water. Important for long flights.
- ❑ Exercise clothing-(Don't make the excuse…Oh I forgot my workout clothes again!)
- ❑ Running shoes and socks
- ❑ Shorts that double as swim trunks, running bra for women
- ❑ Appropriate weather gear. Overcoat, gloves, warm-up suit, hat, etc. Check www.weatherchannel.com for information on the city you are visiting.

How to pack

Place individual items of clothing (i.e., suit, shirts, slacks) in the dry cleaners' plastic bags. This is a great trick, because your clothes will resist wrinkling and the thin plastic lining doesn't take up as much space as a garment bag.

Fill your shoes with rolled socks, small underwear, and other easily misplaced items, and place running shoes in a plastic shopping bag. This will help prevent soiling your clothes with dirty shoes.

What to pack it in

Packing correctly can be a great time saver. Roll-on bags that fit in the overhead compartments work really well. Try to carry everything with you to avoid waiting for your bag, or even worse, losing it. You can save between 20 and 30 minutes of waiting by the luggage carousel if you can fit everything in one bag and avoid having to check baggage. If your bag is so large that you cannot fit it in the overhead compartments, you're going to have issues. The allotted overhead space for most airlines is 9" height X 14"deep X 22" wide. There are lots of great roll-on bags. One ideal bag is the TUMMI 20 carry-on. It's a perfect size for the overhead compartment (8.5" X 13.75" X 20"), and has a zip-out suit compartment and two small, zippered compartments to leave the main packing area free and roomy. You can find them at: http://www.tumi.com/. You can also pick up a beautiful roll-on bag, with the exact same dimensions for a lot less money at a Sam's Warehouse club.

Most traditional briefcases are no longer functional. Today most briefcases need to accommodate a computer and its accessories as well as the traditional paperwork, airline ticket, pens, pencils, etc. A functional replacement for the rectangular and inflexible briefcase is the all-purpose shoulder bag. The bag is not like your father's beautiful leather-bound briefcase; instead it looks like the kind originally used by those wild bicycle messengers. Those messengers had to ride through the rain and sleet and needed a bag durable enough to deliver the bag's contents intact. Here is a list of bags I've researched:

1. **Brenthaven,** Center Load, $69, 800-803-7225, www.brethaven.com

    •   My favorite bag. It's practical yet classic, and works well with any business attire. Doubles as a backpack. Light weight and rugged.

    •   Brenthaven offers a lifetime warranty.

2. **CourierWare,** Deluxe Courier Bag, $95, 800-678-2247, www.courierwareusa.com

    •   Has divided central pockets with six additional storage slots, three on the outside and three on the inside.

3. **REI,** Timbuk2, New Dee Dog Bag, $65, 800-426-4840, www.rei.com

    •   Has a waist strap so it stays secure when you ride a bike.

4. **Land's End,** Original Attaché Bag, $49.50 800-356-444, www.landsend.com

    •   Has lots of pockets and an easy-to-pull zipper. Very affordable.

Being prepared for your trip is the best way to avoid or minimize stress. If you're already stressed and need relief, fear not, it can be done. Coping with stress, once it has seized you, is a skill we all can learn relatively easily. Though you may not be able to avoid stress, you can definitely learn the skills to manage it.

Stress-Relief Techniques and Coping Skills

You can minimize negative reactions to stress by taking the holistic approach to health. If you eat a healthy diet and exercise regularly, you will probably relax and sleep more soundly. Exercise and sleep will keep you less "stressed out." While traveling, you simply have to be more aware of those stressors around you and plan on getting out of the "fight or flight" mode periodically. Once stress hits, you have to find a constructive way to deal with it.

Exercise

Regular aerobic exercise is one of the body's best defenses against negative stress, especially while traveling. Try doing some type of exercise that you genuinely enjoy, and approach it with a relaxed frame of mind. Playing a favorite sport while traveling will provide tremendous benefits. Aerobic exercises, walking, running, or swimming will also help reduce the stress in your body. Again, chasing the beer cart on the golf course doesn't count. We will cover specific exercise routines in Chapter Seven.

Prioritizing

The great motivational speaker and planner Dr. Stephan Covey, in his book *The 7 Habits of Highly Effective People*[10] counsels us to "put first things first," meaning give the highest priority to the most important things in your life. Give the demands and activities of your schedule a priority rating. That way, you can focus on what needs to be done now from your "to do" list and make sufficient time to do those things. Make sure to avoid focusing only on problems.

A little vacation every day

If you have a chance, after or between appointments, schedule some time to yourself or with a colleague and act like a tourist. If you're visiting a new city, research some of the tourist hot spots. Acting like the

---

[10] Dr. Stephan Covey, *The 7 Habits of Highly Effective People*, (New York, NY: Simon & Schuster, 1989), 145.

tourist will provide adventure and show you sides of a city you thought you knew, when, in fact, your familiarity with the city was based only on the airport and your hotel. Visit a museum, a park, or a historical site that you've read up on. Do whatever tourists do just for an hour or two, and that adventure will reduce your stress level and make for a more pleasant trip.

When you plan your business appointments and schedule your priorities, make sure to allow some flexibility. You should try to be as effective and efficient as you can. Don't try to schedule appointments too closely together. I know a lot of you are rolling their eyes at this concept. I am *not* advocating inefficient use of your time. I am suggesting, however, that you try to optimize your time and be smart about what side of town your appointments are on. Remember Murphy's Law: what can go wrong will go wrong. Scheduling, planning, and prioritizing will keep Mr. Murphy at bay.

Good Nutrition

Caffeine, refined sugars, and foods that are high in saturated fats are usually linked to a lifestyle that carries the burden of other stress-filled patterns. Try to eat well while traveling. Skip the fast food places and try to have a few sit-down meals.

Meditation

Does the word meditation make you think of monks chanting and swaying? Meditation can help us all. Meditation is an ancient source of stress release; it triggers deep relaxation and clarity of mind. Some experts recommend 20 minutes a day. Others suggest simply meditating by breathing slowly for a few minutes to break a stressful pattern. Most importantly, meditation means taking time for you to refresh your mind.

How do you meditate?

Many people who meditate find it best to meditate in a sitting position so as to remain alert and not fall asleep (unless, of course falling asleep is your intent). Sit on a cushion so that your pelvis is tilted slightly forwards. Try, if you can, always to meditate in the same place in your room. While traveling, try to use the same position while meditating. Hang the "Do not disturb" card on your door, unplug the phone for a while, and dim the lights. When you start mediating, try to minimize the distractions. With practice, you'll find you can meditate even with some distractions going on around you.

In the beginning, try to meditate for 15 minutes. If you can't make it that long, build yourself up from 5 to 10 minutes. At the end of your meditation, you may want to repeat or simply think about something important that has been on your mind. Once you have cleared your mind, you can often find solutions to problems that are bothering you.

The most commonly used form of breathing that helps one meditate is called Zen Breath. Okay…I used the *Zen* word. Please don't go running off thinking, "this 'Zen thing' is too exotic for me to try." Believe me, if it works for Joe Sixpack, it can work for you.

Zen Breath Counting

The Zen breathing technique is one of the simplest and most effective forms of meditation.

- Sit comfortably and close your eyes. Sit upright because you're not trying to go to sleep. (If you lay down you will probably fall asleep.)

- Become aware of your breathing, but don't change it.

- Listen to your breathing come in, listen to it go out, and count "one." Count "two" on the next exhale, and so on up to 10. Then begin again at one. Try not to change your breathing pattern or anticipate the number to come.

- If you lose count, start over.

Be patient with your initial attempts at meditation. At first, you may feel frustrated or restless, your mind may wander, and you may lose count. Don't worry, you will get better at it. After you get comfortable with this breathing exercise, you'll be able to do it at just about any time and place. You can try it while waiting for your car pool or the train, or for your spouse to get out of the bathroom. You will find that this form of meditation helps you reduce your stress level. This simple breathing technique will allow you to let go of the negative thoughts and worries that create and foster mental and physical tension. It also induces the relaxation response, which has many physical and psychological benefits. Try this technique once or twice daily. With regular practice (like anything you practice), you will increase your meditation capabilities and you will see the rewards.

Acupressure (http://www.healingspirit.com/acupressure.html)

Meditation is not the only Eastern practice you can use to improve your health. Acupuncture and chiropractic medicine have been widely accepted in the United States for years. If allowing someone to stick tiny needles in your body does not appeal to you, there is a less invasive therapy. For those little everyday travel-related stress pains, acupressure can provide effective relief. Since business travelers probably won't have the time or opportunity to visit someone skilled in the art of acupressure, here are some techniques you can perform on yourself. Keep in mind that you can use these techniques throughout the day in the airplane, at the hotel, or just about anywhere.

Breathing and Pressure

For all of the following self-help techniques, use firm pressure. Hold the pressure and breathe deep, relaxed breaths for between four to six counts, until you start to feel some relief.

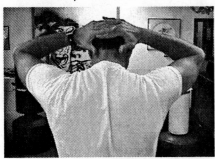

Tension Headaches

Clasp your fingers behind your head and press your thumbs up under the bone where your neck meets your head.

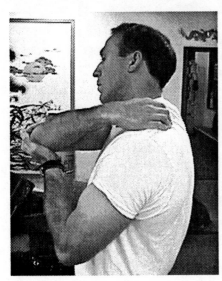

Neck Ache

Hold your right elbow with your left hand, placing your right hand on your left shoulder. Press in with your fingers and the heel (base) of your hand. Squeeze along the top of the shoulder and the side of the neck, toward the back of the neck and under the ear. While you continue to support your elbow, go all the way down between the shoulder blade and the spine, pressing your fingers and releasing. Repeat on the other side.

Pain Relief

Place your right thumb near the top of the fleshy mound between your left thumb and index finger. Place your right index finger opposite your thumb and feel around for the nerve-like sensation. When you've found it squeeze and hold. Repeat on the other hand. Try to relax the other parts of your body when doing this exercise.

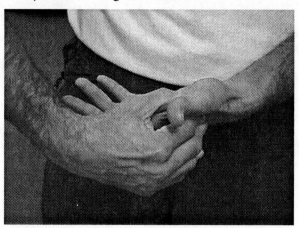

Foot Fatigue

You're going to have to do this one barefoot or with your socks on, so make sure you find an appropriate place. On an airplane some people may take offense if you have feet that smell worse than week-old fish. Cross your legs, place your ankle on your knee. Put one thumb on top of the other and press into the ball of your foot. Hold for one or two breaths, release, and move in half-inch increments down the midline of the foot toward the heel. Now, separate your thumbs and line them up with your second and fourth toes. Draw another line of presses down to the heel. Move your thumbs below the big and little toes and repeat.

Then grab each toe, circle it left and right and give it a gentle tug. Repeat on the other foot.

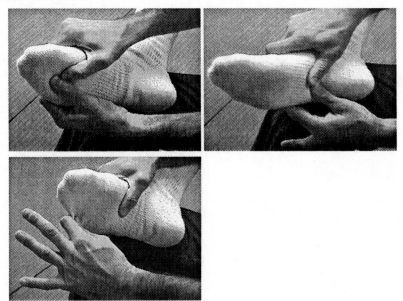

Massage (http://www.doubleclickd.com/theramassage.html)

Many people are aware that massages feel good and relieve stress. Massage also plays a beneficial role in both strength training and flexibility training. Massaging a muscle, or a group of muscles, immediately prior to performing stretching or strength exercises for those muscles, has some of the following benefits:

- **Increased blood flow.** The massaging of the muscles helps to warm-up those muscles, increasing their blood flow and improving their circulation.

- **Relaxation of the massaged muscles.** The massaged muscles are more relaxed. This is particularly helpful when you are about to stretch those muscles. It can also help relieve painful muscle cramps.

- **Removal of metabolic waste.** The massaging action, and the improved circulation and blood flow that results, helps to remove waste products, such as lactic acid, from the muscles. This is a useful practice for relieving post-exercise soreness. You can probably work the knots out of your legs and shoulders. A full body massage, however, is fantastic way to relieve tension. So if you have the opportunity to get to a certified masseuse, be sure to take advantage.

Laughter as Stress Relief

You know, it's almost impossible to feel upset or sad when you're laughing. Try this exercise. Put a big smile on your face, look in the mirror, and say, "I am sad." It doesn't work, does it? Laughing is a physiological response to a happy mental state. Humor helps to make us feel good physically and when we laugh, it's almost impossible to feel bad. One of the best ways to deal with stress and forget about what ails us is to have a good belly laugh.

Humor usually involves some twist of life's normal circumstances. Comedians make us think of common events in new, unrealistic, or ironic ways. They may show us that our day-to-day life shouldn't be taken too seriously, and that we can't take ourselves too seriously. Laughing about life helps us to feel alive and may positively influence our health.

In recent years, scientists have suggested that laughter can have a good effect on the immune system. It's been shown that people who laugh often activate the body's defenses against disease. Obviously, laughter is good for your mental health; it's difficult to stay angry, sad, or stressed out when you're laughing.

Humor will help the business traveler reduce stress and make the trip much more satisfying and enjoyable. We all like to be around people who make us laugh, so make yourself laugh! We don't want to make laughing a new task; hopefully, we all remember how to laugh. We just have to *try* to laugh—let it go when appropriate and whenever you have the chance. Practice laughing with some of the following activities:

- ❑ Read a funny book
- ❑ Read the comics in the newspaper
- ❑ Watch a funny movie
- ❑ Go to a comedy club
- ❑ Listen to comedy recording (headsets for the plane or purchased cassette)
- ❑ Do an Internet search for "humor"
- ❑ Share a funny e-mail with a friend
- ❑ Go to a pet store and play with a puppy or kitten
- ❑ Try to tell a joke or ask someone to tell you their favorite joke

If you need a joke, check out the following websites: http://laugh-a-lot.com/, http://www.baloneymobile.com/29jokes2.html, and http://www.cleanjokes.net/. There are hundreds of humor Web sites out there, so have at it.

Travel Humor

The following are some actual humorous statements made by airline flight crews.

Occasionally, airline attendants make an effort to make the in-flight safety lecture a bit more entertaining. Here are some real examples that have been heard or reported:

- • "As we prepare for takeoff, please make sure your tray tables and seat backs are fully upright in their most uncomfortable position."

- "There may be 50 ways to leave your lover, but there are only 4 ways out of this airplane."

- "Your seat cushions can be used for floatation, and in the event of an emergency water landing, please take them with our compliments."

- "We do feature a smoking section on this flight; if you must smoke, contact a member of the flight crew and we will escort you to the wing of the airplane."

- "Smoking in the lavatories is prohibited. Any person caught smoking in the lavatories will be asked to leave the plane immediately."

Have fun! That's an order! *Ha!*

Chapter Six

Eating & Drinking

Everyone has a love/hate relationship with food. I can't think of single person I know who doesn't, at some time or another, crave something to eat that is "not good" for us. What is it that you crave? What food do you desire while on the road traveling? Is it a juicy T-bone steak, fudge-covered Oreos, or the jelly-filled donut from the bakery on your way to the airport? Try something novel and anti-fitness establishment—*eat it*. Go ahead and plan to partake in what you desire most. Give in to the devil's food cake temptation. I hear loud screams of yes, yes, YES! Do partake, but the key is to do so in moderation. You knew there had to be a catch here.

Plan on "going astray" for a meal or two while you are traveling. If you are going to blow your sensible eating habits, *plan* it. If you have a craving for "death by chocolate" cake for dessert, eat half of a normal portion. Split it with a friend or business associate. When eating a nice meal, remember: **you do not have to clean your plate (like your Mother used to tell you).** It may have been important to eat all the calories possible when you were eight years old, but as adults we can (and should) chose how much we consume. Here are some other tips for eating sensibly at a restaurant or while traveling:

- Eat lean. Take the skin off the chicken and cut the fat off your steak. Also, watch out for garlic butter on your steak. It tastes great, but adds a *huge* amount of fat.

- Eat raw fruits and vegetables. Raw vegetables and fresh fruits contain a maximum amount of vitamins in their natural state that's usually lost when cooked.

- Reduce (or skip!) the butter or margarine.

- Reduce the amount of salad dressing you consume. Try this trick: the next time you order a salad, order your dressing on the side. Before you take a forkful of salad, dip your fork in the dressing, then spear your salad. You will have the taste of the dressing without consuming the calories. It literally will reduce your calories from dressing by 50 percent or more.

- Avoid fried foods. The frying grease is loaded with calories and may make you feel sick. Furthermore, your stomach has a hard time digesting the lard or oil usually used to fry foods. Try eating grilled or baked foods instead.

- Eat slowly. By pacing yourself, you'll enjoy your food more and help your digestive system. If you eat too quickly, you'll "fool" your body into thinking that you're not full yet and continue to eat. Taking your time helps the body to know when to say "when."

- Try to eat smaller meals more often. If you can eat four or five small meals when you're hungry during the day, you are less likely to "pig out" in the evening. Even if you can eat an apple or non-fat yogurt, it will stave off your hunger until dinnertime.

- Eat a variety of foods.

- Don't eat because you are bored.

Prepare Your Meal

Dreading your high-fat, salty, overcooked airline meal? You don't have to settle for it! Call your airline and ask about special meals. All major airlines offer dietary alternatives, as long as these meals are ordered in advance. You can usually choose from low-fat, cold seafood, fruit, or vegetarian alternatives.

Eat and Drink Before You Start the Trip

Eat well before you begin traveling. If you start your trip hungry, you'll wind up at the airport snackatorium, chowing down anything available. If, however, you eat a good healthy meal before you start your trip, you are less likely to be tempted by the wonderfully fatty delicious fresh-baked cookies waiting for you at the airport food court.

Hydrate yourself before your trip. Throughout your travels, remember to drink plenty of water. Sodas, on the other hand, do *not* quench thirst. In fact, most sodas are diuretics, which cause your body to rid itself of fluid. Consuming alcohol will dehydrate your body even faster. If you need a refreshing thirst quencher, try mixing apple juice and sparkling water. Try a 50 percent apple juice and a 50 percent water mix and adjust to your tastes. It will quench your thirst and provide a dose of vitamin C.

I Really Want to Lose Fat Weight!

There are numerous scientific diets out there; I see them advertised every other week. This or that "noted expert" will talk about how to lose weight. Many of these "diet leaders" have had tremendous followings based on little more than good looks or shallow popularity. There is no doubt: there are many diet industry experts who do know exactly how to reduce your weight. Your question should be, "How do I stick to my selected type of diet while traveling?"

How can you be successful in losing weight? Most health experts will tell you that "diets" by themselves typically don't work long term. Strict diets based on starvation or on military-style discipline usually have a backlash effect. That backlash is usually in the form of ravenous hunger, a low energy level, and hunger-induced insomnia. The best type of diet allows you to retain your energy level through the right combination of carbohydrates, proteins, and fats.[11] Yes, fat. Fat is necessary to any healthy diet; it's the fuel that feeds muscles. Monounsaturated fats, which come from olive oil and avocados, are easily digested by your system. Polyunsaturated fats, like those from vegetable oil or animal-based products are harder to digest and are stored in your body. Keep in mind that there are three types of fats—saturated, unsaturated, and monounsaturated—and you should be eating roughly equal proportions of them all. The bad fats (saturated fats, and for some people polyunsaturated fats) are in foods like hydrogenated oils (hydrogenation, as its name implies, is the process of adding a hydrogen atom to oil to make it a solid, saturated fat). For more information on fats, try this link: http://www.fatassassins.com/noframes/food.html.

Remember: the weight scale does not tell the entire story. Muscle is heavier than fat. Fat loss is more important than weight loss. You lose fat by expending more calories than you take in. For the average business traveler, we eat when we have time or as part of business and social events. So how do we keep a watch on and a move toward fat reduction? Here are some tips:

1. Keep a record of what you eat for a week. Look at the labels for fat content and calories. Listed below is a calorie chart of foods we normally eat. Try to become aware of what, when, and how much you eat. Typically, weight-conscious individuals tend to starve themselves all day, only to "pig out" at night. You will be more successful if you consume the bulk of your calories during the day, thereby preventing those late-night hunger pangs and sluggishness. When you get hungry at night, you're inclined to care less about your diet and more about having a full belly.

---

[11] Michael A. Schmidt, *Smart Fats*, (Berkeley, CA: North Atlantic Books, 1997).

2. The second step is to examine your list and make choices as to what junk food you can cut back on or eliminate entirely. For instance, a can of cola or a candy bar can have up to 240 calories! Try drinking only half of the can, or share the cola by pouring the other six ounces into a cup full of ice and giving it to your buddy. The same goes for junk food—if you're going to have a candy bar, try to split it. Use the same approach to your eating. Do you need extra sauce on that steak? Can you make do with a smaller portion? Most restaurants will allow ordering smaller portions; just ask.

3. Next, measure your waistline (for men) and your hips (for women). Take measurements at the beginning of your health regimen. If you're maintaining your weight and your waist/hip size shrinks even slightly, you're probably reducing your overall body fat.

4. Finally, review your eating records. Look at the food you have reduced or eliminated from your diet, then measure your waist/hipline.

Success Tips

- Be committed to a new lifestyle of health and fitness.

- Take charge; assert yourself and your program.

- Be responsible for nutritious meals and regular exercise.

- Develop a plan for fitness and stick with it daily.

- Reward yourself with something other than food, like a new tie or blouse.

- Enjoy and savor the results: feeling better, looking better, having more vitality.

Caloric Chart of Fast Food Restaurants

Name of Restaurant / Food Item	Calories[12]
Arby's	
Beef 'n Cheddar	508
Broccoli and Cheddar Baked Potato	417
Chicken Breast Sandwich	445
Giant Roast Beef	544
Grilled Chicken Deluxe	430
French Fries:	
Cheddar Fries (small)	399
Curly Fries (small)	337
Light Chicken Deluxe Sandwich	276
Light Roast Beef Deluxe	294
Light Roast Turkey Deluxe	260
Regular Roast Beef	383
Roast Beef Sub	623
Salads:	
Garden Salad	117
Chef Salad	205
Chicken Salad	204
Salad Dressings (per packet):	
Blue Cheese	295
Ranch	349
French	322
1000 Island	298
Light Italian	23

---

[12] http://gourmetconnection.com/ezine/calorie/cfast.shtml

Burger King

Apple Pie	369
BK Broiler Chicken Sand. (no mayo)	267
BK Broiler Sauce	37
Burgers:	
Bacon Cheeseburger	510
Bacon Cheeseburger Deluxe	584
Cheeseburger	317
Double Cheeseburger	483
Hamburger	275
Hamburger Deluxe	344
Whopper	614
Whopper w/ cheese	709
Double Whopper	844
Double Whopper w/ cheese	935
Whopper Jr.	322
Whopper Jr. w/ cheese	364
Chicken Sandwich	685
Chicken Tenders (6 piece)	236
Crossan'wich:	
Bacon, egg, cheese	355
Ham, egg, cheese	351
Sausage, egg, cheese	534
French Fries (regular)	372
French Toast Sticks	538
Hash Browns	215
Ocean Catch Fish Fillet Sand.	479
Onion Rings (regular)	339
Pies:	
Cherry	360
Lemon	290

Salads:

Chef Salad	178
Chunky Chicken Salad	142
Garden Salad	95

Scrambled Egg Platter:

	549
w/ bacon	610
w/sausage	768

Shakes:

Chocolate	326
Vanilla	334

Whaler Sandwich:

	488
with cheese	530

Domino's Pizza

12" Pizza (2 slices):

Cheese	360
Deluxe	540
Extravaganza	510
Pepperoni	410
Pepperoni, sausage, mushrooms	460
Sausage	430
Vegi Feast	390

Kentucky Fried Chicken (KFC)

Buttermilk Biscuit	235
Chicken Littel Sand.	169
Cole Slaw (1 serving)	114
Colonel's Chicken Sand.	482

Fried Chicken:

Extra Crispy:

Breast	344
Drumstick	205

Thigh	415
Wing	230
Original Recipe:	
Breast	276
Drumstick	150
Thigh	290
Wing	181
Fried Chicken Dinners:	
Original Recipe (drumstick/thigh)	643
Extra Crispy (drumstick/thigh)	765
French Fries	244
Kentucky Nuggets (6 piece)	280

McDonald's

Apple Pie	260
Big Mac	570
Bacon, egg, cheese Biscuit	483
Biscuit w/ sausage, egg	585
Cheeseburger	318
Chef Salad	170
Chicken McNuggets (6 piece)	323
Danish-Apple	390
Egg McMuffin	340
Filet o Fish	435
Fries-Large	400
Hamburger	263
Hash Browns	144
Hotcakes w/ syrup & Butter	500
McChicken	490
McDLT	680
McLean Deluxe	320
Quarter Pounder w/ cheese	525

Sausage McMuffin	427
Scrambled Eggs	180
Shake-Chocolate	383
Strawberry Sundae	320

Pizza Hut
Medium Pizzas, 2 slices:

Hand-tossed Pizza:	
Cheese	518
Pepperoni	500
Supreme	540
Pan Pizza:	
Cheese	492
Pepperoni	540
Supreme	589
Personal Pan Pizza (1 pizza):	
Pepperoni	675
Supreme	647
Thin 'n Crispy Pizza:	
Cheese	398
Pepperoni	413
Supreme	459

Taco Bell
Burritos:

Bean	447
Beef	493
Chicken	334
Combo	407
Supreme	503
Chilito	383
Guacamole (2 tbsp.)	34

Mexi Melt:
 Beef   266
 Chicken   257
Nacho Cheese Sauce (2 tbsp.)   103
Nachos (1 order):
 BellGrande   649
 Regular   346
 Supreme   367
Salsa (1 serving)   18
Soft Taco:
 Chicken   213
 Supreme   272
Taco   183
Taco Supreme   230
Taco Salad   905
Tostada   243

Wendy's

Baked Potato, plain   250
 Bacon/cheese   510
 Broccoli/cheese   450
 Cheese   550
 Chili/cheese   600
 Sour cream/chives   500
Big Classic Sand.   570
Breaded Chicken Sand.   450
Chicken Club Sand.   520
Cheeseburgers:
 Double   590
 Jr. Cheeseburger   320
 Jr. Deluxe   390
 Jr. w/ bacon   440

Chicken Nuggets (6 piece)	280
Chili-large	290
Cole Slaw (1/2 cup)	90
Country Fried Steak Sand.	460
Fish Sand.	460
French Fries-Large	450
Frost Dairy Dessert-large	578
Grilled Chicken Sand.	290
Hamburgers:	
Hamburger	350
with everything	440
Double hamburger	520
Jr. Burger	270
Kids Meal	270
Salads:	
Caesar	160
Deluxe Garden, no dressing	110
Grilled chicken, no dressing	200
Side, no dressing	60
Taco, no dressing	640

Category & Food Item	Caloric Content[13]
Beverages	
Beer:	
Regular, 12oz.	150
Light, 12oz.	100

---

[13] http://gourmetconnection.com/ezine/calorie/cstore.shtml

Gin, rum,vodka,whiskey-1.5oz.	95-110
Wine, table-3.5oz.	140
Carbonated Beverages, 12oz.:	
Club soda	0
Cola	160
Ginger-ale	125
Lemon-lime	150
Orange, grape	180
Cocoa:	
Hershey's w/ 2% milk (6oz.)	135
Swiss Miss w/ water (1pkg)	110
Coffee:	
Cappuccino w/ whole milk (12oz.)	296
Espresso (2.4oz.)	0
Latte (16oz.)	
whole milk, grated chocolate	350

Dairy and Eggs

Butter – regular:	
1 tbsp.	100
1 stick	813
Butter – Whipped:	
1 tbsp.	67
1 stick / 1/2 cup	542
Cheese (1 oz.):	
American	106
Blue	100
Bonbel (Laughing Cow)	70
Brie	90
Cheddar	114
Cottage (1/2 cup) 4%	110
Cottage (1/2 cup) 1%	90

Cream Cheese (1 tbsp.)	52
Feta (1 oz.)	75
Monterey (1oz.)	106
Mozzarella (1oz.):	
whole milk	80
part skim	72
Parmesan (1 tbsp.)	23
Provolone (1oz.)	100
Ricotta (1/2 cup):	
whole milk	216
part skim	171
Swiss (1oz.)	107
Cream, Half & Half, 1 tbsp.	20
Coffee Mate powdered cream (1 tbsp.)	30
Sour cream (2 tbsp.)	60
Whipped Cream-Reddi Whip (2 tbsp.)	20
Milk (1 cup):	
1%	104
2%	121
Buttermilk	99
Chocolate, 2% milk	179
Skim	86
Low Fat Yogurt (8oz.):	
Breyers	250
Columbo	120
Dannon	210
Dannon Fruit on Bottom	240
Yoplait (6oz.)	170
Non-Fat Yogurt (8oz.):	
Columbo, fruit flavors	190
Dannon blended (6oz.)	150-160

Weight Watchers ultimate	90
Yoplait light (6oz.)	90
Eggs-1 egg:	
Large	79
white only	16
yolk only	63
Egg Substitute (1/4 cup):	
Egg beaters	30
Healthy choice	25
Scramblers	35

Fats & Oils

Margarines (1 tbsp.):	
Fleischman's	90
Imperial	90
Land o' Lakes Country Morn	100
Land o' Lakes Light	50
Move Over Butter	90
Promise	90
Shedds Spread, churn style	80
Shedds Spread, spread stick	80
Margarine Tubs:	
Fleischman's	90
I Can't Believe It's Not Butter	70
Parkay spread	60
Promise	90
Promise Ultra	35
Promise Ultra Fat Free	5
Oils (1 tbsp.):	119-120

Canola, coconut, corn, cottonseed, olive, palm,
peanut, safflower, sesame, soybean, sunflower

Salad Dressings (2 tbsp.):

Blue Cheese Wishbone chunky	150
Kraft Free	45
Catalina	
Kraft Free	45
regular Kraft	140
Cole Slaw Dressing, Kraft	150
French, Kraft	120
Honey Dijon, Hidden Valley	35
Italian, Good Seasons	140
Ranch, Kraft Free	50
Ranch, Kraft regular	170

Mayonnaise (1 tbsp.):

Hellmann's Light	50
Hellmann's regular	100
Kraft Free	10
Kraft light	50
Kraft Regular	100
Miracle Whip	70
Miracle Whip Light	40
Shortening, Crisco (1 tbsp.)	110

Frozen, Microwave & Refrigerated Foods

Waffles (2):

Aunt Jemima Buttermilk	170
Eggo's Buttermilk	220
NutraGrain Eggo	180
Dinty Moore Stew, canned 1 cup	230
Hormel Chili, no beans, 1 cup	360
Lean Cuisine (1 package)	180-290
Mrs. Paul's Breaded Fish Fillets (1)	170

Swanson Hungry Man:

Chicken or Beef Pot Pie	620
Fried Chicken	810

Tyson (1 meal):

Blackened Chicken	270
Chicken Marsala	180
Honey Roasted Chicken	220

Weight Watchers (1 meal):

Broccoli & Cheese Bkd Potato	230
Cheese Manicotti	260
Italian Cheese Lasagna	300
Stouffer's French Bread Pizza (1)	350
Jeno's pizza (1/2 pizza)	250

Fats in Foods Chart

Fatty Acid Content Of Common Dietary Fats

	Monounsaturated	Saturated	Polyunsaturated	Cholesterol (mg/tbsp)
Olive Oil	77%	14%	9%	0
Canola Oil	62%	6%	32%	0
Margarine	49%	17%	34%	0
Peanut Oil	49%	18%	33%	0
Lard	47%	41%	22%	12
Butter	31%	65%	4%	31
Corn Oil	25%	13%	62%	0
Soybean Oil	24%	15%	61%	0
Sunflower Oil	20%	11%	69%	0

Calculating Fat Content of Food

The percentage of calories from fat in a given food can be calculated as follows:

(Fat grams x 9) ÷ Total Calories * 100 = % Calories from fat.

For example, a McDonald's Big Mac is 562 Calories, and contains 32 grams of fat.

(32 * 9) ÷ 562 * 100 = 51.2% of C

http://www.fatassassins.com/noframes/food.html

Train with your Brain: Activities and their Approximate Hourly Caloric Cost for Different Body Weights

Or: How Much You Burn Is Determined By How Much You Weigh
http://www.mineralconnection.com/train13.htm.

If you weigh…	100	125	150	175	200	225	250	275	300
Light Aerobics	104	154	204	254	304	354	404	454	504
Walking 2.5 mph	104	154	204	254	304	354	404	454	504
Gardening	118	168	218	268	318	368	418	468	518
Golf	145	195	245	295	345	395	445	505	545
Lawn Mowing	145	195	245	295	345	395	445	505	545
Light Calisthenics	172	222	272	322	372	422	472	522	572
Light Weight Training	172	222	272	322	372	422	472	522	572
House Cleaning	172	222	272	322	372	422	472	522	572
Walking 3.75 mph	199	249	299	349	399	449	499	549	599
Swimming .25 mph	199	249	299	349	399	449	499	549	599
Medium Aerobics	240	290	340	390	440	490	540	590	640
Badminton	247	297	347	397	447	497	547	597	947
Wood Chopping	294	344	394	444	494	544	594	644	694

Medium Weight Training	342	392	442	492	542	592	642	692	742
Slow Jogging	376	426	476	526	576	626	676	726	776
Heavy Calisthenics	444	494	544	594	644	694	744	794	844
Heavy Aerobics	444	494	544	594	644	694	744	794	844
Heavy Weight Training	512	562	612	662	712	762	812	862	912
Medium Jogging	512	562	612	662	712	762	812	862	912
Cycling	560	610	660	710	760	810	860	910	960
Fast Jogging	580	630	680	730	780	830	880	910	960

Chapter Seven

Exercise While Traveling

Phone Ahead

Call your hotel before you go on the trip. Ask about workout facilities either on-site or nearby. Ask about parks, running tracks, hiking trails, golf, swimming, or whatever interests you. Knowing what is available will help you decide on the clothing and shoes you might want to pack.

Get an Airport Workout

Until the death of Nicole Simpson and the "trial of the century," O.J. Simpson was known as the athlete who could sprint through airports. You don't need to follow in O.J.'s footsteps, but you can still use the airport terminal to fit in some exercise. Airport delays are frustrating and stressful. Don't go to the burger joint or pizza place and pig out to pass the time. Use the airport terminal as a place to get your exercise by walking or speed walking. Change into your athletic shoes, store your carry-on in a locker (or have your sedentary friend watch your bags), and go for a brisk walk. Any amount of walking will exercise your legs and make you feel energized.

The Difficulty Could Be Just in Getting Started

Get into the Exercise Groove

Exercise will jumpstart your entire health effort, yet for many of us, *starting* seems to be the most difficult part. Despite knowing how beneficial a regular exercise routine would be for them, many people are not exercising at sufficient levels to impact their health—especially while on the road. We hear countless messages each week extolling the physical and mental virtues of working out regularly. From infomercials to athletic shoe ads, everybody is encouraged to do some form of exercise! So why aren't we exercising if we know it's good for us?

The most common excuses I hear are **lack of time** and **lack of energy**. We all could find the time if health and fitness were part of our overall mission and goals. Excuses, in the business world, are rarely tolerated; the financial numbers and results matter above all else. The same type of attitude can be applied to your travel fitness regime. Businesspeople learn not to provide or accept excuses, so let's try to work through some typical excuses.

Overcoming the "Not Enough Time" Excuse

We all wish there were 25 hours in the day. That extra hour would help us take care of the things we need to, like our health. Time is a finite dimension in a world of infinite opportunities, thus, it may help to shift your priorities. In order to make fitness a reality, you have to make your exercise regime one of your top priorities.

One way to make fitness a top priority is to start your day off with exercise. If you start your day with an exercise routine, you are more likely to stick with it. The rest of your day will be invigorated by morning exercise.

Overcoming the "Not Enough Energy" Excuse

Make the first step towards increasing your energy level. "Lack of energy" is not a viable excuse. Your energy level is raised as you exercise, so waiting to have more energy to exercise is a backward approach. It's like waiting for the motor of your car to burn up before you can add oil. Increase your physical activity and you'll build more vitality into your overall lifestyle.

Need Motivation?

It's tough to stay motivated and to exercise, especially when traveling around the country or the world. The temptations *not* to do anything about your health are everywhere. How can you consistently exercise when the only consistent thing in life is change?

Look back and review your mission statement and your goals weekly. What goals did you write down to entice you to be more active? If you didn't write it down, do it now. Are your goals to feel healthier? To have more energy? To look slimmer? To have more strength? Be prepared for your priorities to change occasionally, but remember your written mission and goals/objectives, then get back on track and stay focused.

The Ideal Workout (If You Have the Time)

Now that you have reviewed your mission and goals, you should be in the right frame of mind to get going. We are all looking to have the ideal workout. The ideal workout means everything is perfect: you have the time, the weather is great, you feel like working out, and you have an ideal exercise facility.

Though you may not ever be able to find the ideal scenario to work out, you should try to perform the ideal workout. The ideal workout consists of three groups of exercises, which should be completed in the following sequence:

1. Warm-up and stretching
2. The workout itself:
   a. cardiovascular
   b. strength
3. Cool down and stretching

The Warm-Up and Stretching

Warming up is quite literally the process of increasing your core body temperature. Stretching alone is *not* a warm-up; it's only one part of the process. A proper warm-up is divided into three phases:

1. general warm-up

2. stretching

3. sport-specific activity

It is very important that you perform the general warm-up *before* you stretch. It is *not* a good idea to attempt to stretch before your muscles are warm. **Not warming up can greatly increase your risk of injury.**

It is important to note that active stretches and isometric stretches should *not* be part of your warm-up because they are often counterproductive. The goals of the warm-up should be: a) an improved elasticity, and b) reduction of potential injury to the muscles.

The general warm-up is divided into two parts: 1) joint rotations, and 2) aerobic activity. These two activities should be performed in the order specified above. The general warm-up should begin with joint rotations. This activity facilitates joint motion by lubricating the entire joint with synovial fluid, a lubricating fluid secreted by certain membranes. It's kind of like 10W-40 for your joints; it helps get the creaks out. This lubrication permits your joints to function more easily when called upon to work in an activity. You should perform slow circular movements, both clockwise and counter-clockwise, until the joint seems to move smoothly. You should rotate joints in the following order (or in reverse order):

1. wrists

2. elbows

3. shoulders

4. neck

5. trunk/waist
6. hips
7. legs
8. knees
9. ankles

Aerobic Activity Warm-Up

Once you have completed the joint rotation exercises, you need to raise your core body temperature and get your blood pumping. You can increase your body temperature by slow aerobic activities such as jumping rope or jogging in place. The increase in blood flow in your muscles will improve your flexibility and reduce the potential for injury. Here are some additional aerobic activities that are ideal for warm-up:

- Squat thrusts
- Mountain climbers
- Knee bends
- Jumping jacks

Stretching is critical for every fitness activity. Many people neglect this part of their workout and wonder why they are sore or injury prone all the time. Stretching will increase your flexibility and significantly reduce your chances of pulling or tearing muscles. It will also improve your performance. A flexible muscle reacts and contracts faster than a non-flexible muscle. Flexibility also increases your agility and balance. Stretching exercises should be performed after a short warm-up, between weightlifting sets, and/or during your cool down. As an added benefit, stretching is an excellent relaxation technique. Use your stretching time to focus on your sport or workout, visualizing success.

Stretching Phase of the Warm-Up

The stretching phase of your warm-up should consist of two parts:

1. stationary stretching, and

2. dynamic stretching.

Stationary stretches should be performed *before* any dynamic stretches in your warm-up. Performing static stretches first will help you reduce the possibility of injury. Once you have completed your general warm-up, your muscles will feel warmer and more elastic. Immediately following your general warm-up, you should engage in some slow, relaxed, stationary stretching. Start with your back, followed by your upper body, then lower body. Perform these stretches in an unhurried and relaxed manner, stretching your muscles in the order listed below.

The following is a list of stretching exercises you can incorporate into your workout. Hold each stretch for 10 to 15 seconds and do not bounce. Breathe deeply during the stretch.

Neck Rotation

Turn your head to the side, stretching your chin toward your shoulder. Then turn your head back to center and repeat to the other side.

Forearm Stretch

Extend your right arm straight out in front of you with your palm downward. With the left hand, grasp the fingers of the right hand and pull back gently, stretching the wrist and forearm. Repeat with the left arm.

Triceps Stretch

Raise one arm straight up, so your upper arm is near your ear. Bend at the elbow and let your hand fall to the back of your neck. With the other arm, reach behind your head and place your hand on top of the bent elbow. Gently pull down and back on the elbow. Repeat with the other arm.

Trunk Stretch

Stand with your feet a little more than shoulder-width apart. Reach your left arm overhead and bend to the right at the waist. Repeat on the opposite side.

Torso Twist

Stand at arm's length from the wall, with the wall at your side. Reach one arm out and place your hand on the wall. Reach the other arm around the body, stretching the hand to the wall. Repeat on the opposite side.

Chest Stretch

Stand with your feet shoulder-width apart. Clasp your hands behind your back and gently press your arms upward, keeping your arms straight.

Back Stretch

Lie on your back and bring one knee to your chest. Hold the knee with both hands and gently pull in. Alternate knees and repeat.

Hip Roll

Lie on your back and bend your knees, with your feet flat on the floor. Let your knees fall to the right while reaching both arms across your body to the left. Hold the stretch, then roll your hips over to the left, stretching your arms to the right, and repeat the stretch.

Lower Back Reach

Sit on the floor with your legs straight out in front of you. Reach forward toward your toes, keeping your chin up and lower back slightly arched. Try not to round your back or tuck your chin in; this decreases the effectiveness of the stretch.

Butterfly Stretch

Sit on the floor, bend your knees out to the sides and bring the soles of your feet together. Place your hands on your knees and gently press your knees toward the floor. Keep your back straight.

Lateral Hip Stretch

Sit on the floor with both legs straight in front of you. Bend your left leg and place your left foot over your right knee. Then place your right hand on the outside of the left knee and gently pull the knee toward your right shoulder, twisting the torso to the left, until you feel the stretch in your left hip. Repeat on the opposite side.

Hamstring Stretch

Stand with your legs shoulder-width apart with your left leg slightly in front of your right. Shift your weight to the back leg (the right) and bend the knee, turning the knee and toe to the right. Extend the left leg and place the heel on the floor, toes in the air. Keep your back straight and bend forward at the hips until you feel the stretch in the hamstring of the left leg. Repeat with the opposite leg.

V-Stretch

Sit on the floor with your legs extended to either side so they form a "V". Bend forward, grasp your toes or ankles, and stretch your chest toward the floor. Try to go a little lower each time you perform the stretch.

Leaning Calf Stretch

Stand about two and a half feet from a wall. Place your hands on the wall and lean in, gently pushing your hips forward. Keep your legs straight and your heels flat on the floor.

Quadriceps Stretch

Lie face down and reach back with your right arm to grasp your right ankle. Pull your foot toward your buttocks. Be sure to keep your hips and pelvis on the floor. Repeat with your left leg.

I know what you're thinking: "I don't have time for all this stretching!" Most business travelers do not have a lot of time to stretch all these muscles before a workout. If you don't have the time, stretch those muscles you will use heavily during your planned workout. For instance, if your workout is running, focus on the leg stretches. If your workout is weightlifting or upper body, focus on that area.

Dynamic Warm-Up Stretching

I hear your pleas: "Enough with the stretching already!" Once you have performed your static stretches, you should engage in some light dynamic stretching: leg-raises and arm-swings in all directions. In dynamic stretches, there are no bounces or "jerky" movements. An example of dynamic stretching would be slow, controlled leg swings, arm swings, or torso twists.

At this point you should feel like you're about to start sweating. Don't get fatigued—the workout is about to start.

Sport-Specific Warm-Ups

You should focus the last part of your warm-up on movements that are a "slow motion" or "light" versions of the movements that you will be performing during your athletic activity. For example, if you are going to be playing golf, take a few slow practice swings; if you're going to be lifting weights, lift really light weights to start. Such *sport-specific* activity is beneficial because it improves balance, coordination, and, again, may reduce the risk of injury. See http://www.enteract.com/~bradapp/ docs/rec/stretching/ for details.[14]

The Workout (http://www.fitnesslink.com/exercise.htm)

How to Find 30 Minutes to Work Out

If you've completed your health and fitness goals and objectives and you still can't find the time for exercise, consider what health experts say. The American College of Sports Medicine (ACSM) and the Centers for Disease Control and Prevention (CDC) reviewed the latest research and agree on this basic recommendation: "Every American adult should accumulate 30 minutes or more of moderate-intensity physical activity over the course of most days of the week." Equally important, yet not well understood by the general public, are new research findings about the value of intermittent physical activity. According to these new findings, exercising for a total of 30 minutes a day with several breaks also

---

[14] Copyright © 1993-1998 by Bradford D. Appleton. Permission is granted to make and distribute verbatim copies of this document at no charge or at a charge that covers reproducing the cost of the copies, provided that the copyright notice and this permission notice are preserved on all copies.

increases calorie expenditures and can be an option for those who cannot fit 30 minutes of sustained activity into their schedules.[15]

That's not as tough as it sounds. You can easily accrue your 30 minutes of daily exercise—it does *not* have to be continuous exercise. Aim for at least three 10-minute blocks of daily exercise time. Try something as simple as walking for 10 minutes, marching up and down the stairs for 10 minutes, swimming for 10 minutes, and doing 10 minutes of calisthenics.

The Anderson 30-Minute No-Sweat Workout

After having enrolled my children in a self-defense karate class, I met the owner of Double Action Training Academy, Bob Anderson. Bob turned out to be one of fittest individuals I have ever known—or seen, for that matter. At 6 foot 4 and 220 pounds with 6 percent body fat, he made even those male models from Men's Health and Men's Fitness look like wimps.

I ended up joining his martial arts studio, partially because I was interested in taking ju-jitsu and partially because I wanted to know how this 50 year old stayed fitter then any 20 year old on the planet. Bob had also been a bodyguard and traveled extensively all around the world. As a bodyguard he found himself having to be at his best mentally and physically all the time. He developed a fitness program that can be performed when either no gym is available or you just don't have the time to make it to a gym. As we discussed different aspects of fitness, Bob had

---

[15] According to Steven Blair, P.E.D., Director of the Cooper Institute for Aerobics Research and an advisor to the *Shape Up America!* campaign, "While it was once thought that sustained activity was needed to have a health benefit, increasing evidence now suggests that accumulating 30 minutes of activity over the course of the day also increases caloric expenditure and can be an option for those who cannot fit 30 minutes of sustained activity into their schedules." See http://www.shapeup.org/dated/060195.htm for more details.

me convinced that his workout would function very well for the business traveler. I recruited him to write the exercise portion of this book based on programs he had developed and refined over the last 20 years. He developed programs for advanced, intermediate, and beginner fitness levels, called the Anderson Workout. Not only can it be done in your hotel room, it's an ultimate workout in just 30 to 45 minutes.

Overview

Different people respond differently to any one given program; therefore, not only will we give you sample programs, but we will show you how you can adjust the program so that it is tailor-made for you. After 30 to 45 days, your body chemically adjusts to your program's workload; therefore, you should plan to alter your routine. By changing the tempo, intensity, and amount of reps or sets, your body will be challenged and respond more efficiently, ensuring you continued results.

Without getting into complicated anatomy, you have muscles that are designed to push and muscles that are designed to pull. One school of thought is that pushing muscles should be worked one day, and pulling muscles on the next. The other school of thought is that you should work both pushing and pulling groups of muscles on the same day. Switching it around gives you a good way to adjust your program after that first 30 or 45 days.

Later in this chapter, there is a menu of exercises so you'll be able to choose and change your program. We will show you programs for beginner, intermediate, and advanced levels. First, we will start with a beginner's program. In this program you will exercise every other day. Keep in mind that this program is designed for people who *do not* have an exercise routine to condition the body for more demanding exercise programs to come.

Beginner Program

If you don't currently have an exercise program, this is where you might want to start. To get your body conditioned to exercise, start by working every other day throughout the week doing a full, but light, workout.

Day One:

Chest: Push-ups 10 to 15 reps and two sets.
Back: Push-ups with the hands spread wide, fingers pointed out, weight pushed a little forward. Do 15 reps for two sets.
Shoulders: Incline push-ups. Do 8 to 10 reps for two sets.

Don't get discouraged with all of these push-ups—contrary to what you might be thinking, this is *not* just a push-up program. There are a lot of exciting exercises to come. However, one of the best and quickest ways to get in shape is to lift your own body weight. This is why military specialty groups use this type of callisthenic exercise all the time. Remember: we're talking about a starter program. You're getting the body ready to hit it. Note that if you already have an exercise routine, you may opt to start with the intermediate program.

<u>Arms</u>: Take one of your suitcases, and if it's already empty, fill it with phone books, shoes, etc. to get it to the desired weight. Put one hand on the wall and put your feet back a few paces. Lean forward, and with the other hand on your suitcase, curl it 10 times. Then switch hands and repeat for two sets.

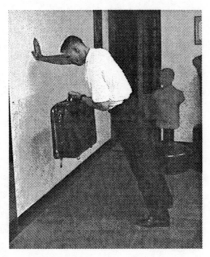

<u>Triceps</u>: These dips are done by putting your hands on a chair and setting your feet on the bed or another chair. Now lower yourself as far as you can. Do 10 reps for two sets.

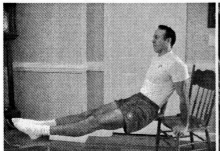 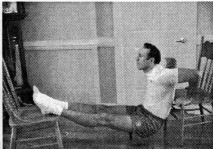

<u>Legs</u>: Put your feet shoulder-width apart, with your toes pointed slightly out. Squat down until your legs are parallel with the ground bottom, then stand up. Do 10 to 15 reps for two sets.

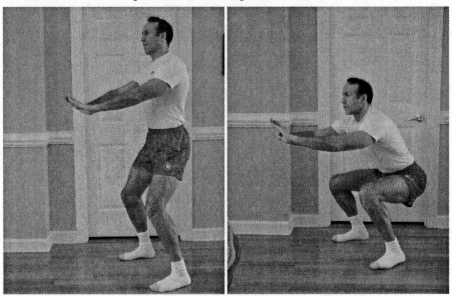

<u>Abs</u>: On your back, with your knees bent and feet on the floor, put your hands on your temples and crunch up until your shoulders and upper back are off the ground. Do 15 reps for one set.

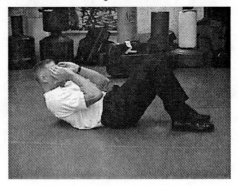

Next are <u>knee presses</u>. While keeping one leg straight and off the ground 6 inches, grab your other shin with both hands and pull your knee up to or as close to your chin as you can. Hold it and count: "One, two, three, *one*, one, two, three, *two*," and so on until you reach 15.

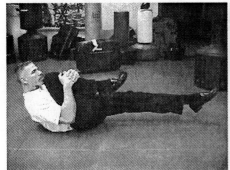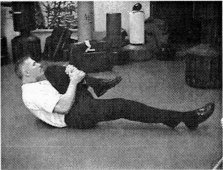

Then, without stopping, do another 15 count, bringing your knee to your chin without the use of your hands. Do one set.

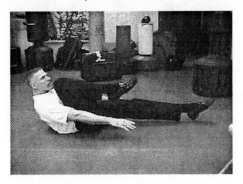

- Do this beginner routine every other day for one week.
- Add one set on to everything but abs for the next week.
- After two weeks of this program you'll be ready for the next level.

Intermediate Program

Starting your third week, we go to the intermediate program. This will be a two day on, one day off routine.

Day One:

<u>Chest:</u> Start with push-ups. Place your hands shoulder-width apart. Put your feet up on a suitcase. Do 10 to 12 repetitions with strict form and a medium tempo. Rest 20 to 30 seconds, then do another set. Do three sets.

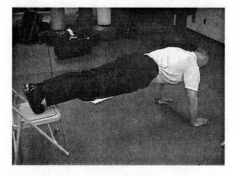

The next exercise is <u>chair dips</u>. Take two chairs, face them back-to-back, and set a pillow in between them. The pillow will cushion your fall just in case your muscles give out, you lose your balance, or the chairs break. (Keep in mind, however, that Bob never had a chair break and he weighs 220 pounds.) Before you use anything in the hotel room for exercise equipment, make sure you check it thoroughly and make sure it will support your weight. If you don't have any weightlifting gloves, you can use two hand towels for cushions. Lay the hand towels on the top of the chairs to make your grip more comfortable. Now you're ready to do chair dips. It's important to keep your chin pressed to your chest as you do the dip as this motion will help you focus on your chest muscles. Make sure you go *all* the way down and *all* the way up. Do 10 reps. Rest 20 to 30 seconds. Do three sets.

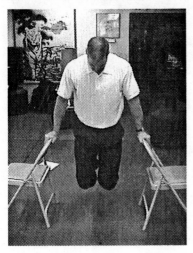 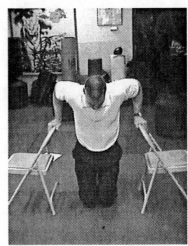

<u>Back</u>: These are pull-ups on the bathroom door. Try using a towel for this exercise—a good thick towel on the top of the door makes for a comfortable grip. Since pulling yourself up will depend on your strength and weight, do as many pull-ups as you can with good form. Rest 20 to 30 seconds. Do three sets.

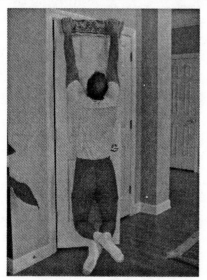 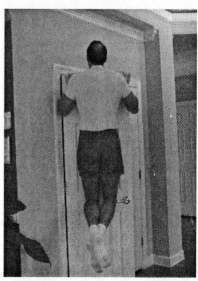

<u>Legs</u>: Squats are one of the best exercises for legs and glutes (butt). Stand in front of a chair with your feet shoulder-width apart, and your toes slightly pointed out. With your arms stretched out in front of you to help you with your balance, squat down until your butt lightly hits the chair. Make sure that your knees do not bend past your toes, then stand up. Do 10 reps for three sets.

Next are <u>lunges</u>. Put your hands on your hips, step forward with your left foot, and squat down until the knee of your right leg is about an inch off the ground. Now rise immediately and repeat, making sure that your knee doesn't touch the ground on the way down. Do 10 reps on each side for three sets.

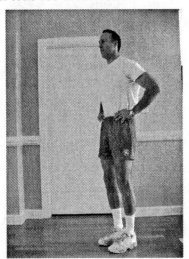 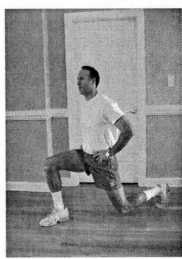

<u>Abs</u>: Do 15 crunches.

Next do 15 knee presses. While lying on your back with your knees bent, cross your left foot over your right knee, and put your right hand on your temple. Then crunch up, touching your right elbow to your left knee, then moving back down. Do 15 on one side then 15 on the other. Do all three exercises in quick succession without resting.

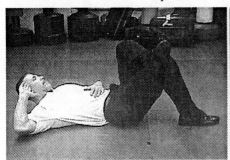 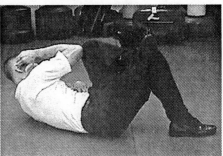

Guess what sports fans? We've finished our first day.

Day Two:

<u>Shoulders and Arms</u> (biceps, triceps, and forearms): We'll start by "super-setting" the biceps and triceps. Super-setting means that you will do an exercise for two different muscles in succession without stopping. Now, grab one of your suitcases and fill it with a phone book, water bottles, shoes, etc. until it reaches your desired weight. Then put one hand on the wall, lean over, and slowly curl the suitcase up. Do 10 reps, then change hands and repeat.

Without resting, go to a table or counter and do <u>triceps dips</u>. Put your hands together, your feet back, and dip down, keeping your elbows pointed toward the ground. Go under (or to) the edge of the table or counter. Do 10 reps and repeat for three cycles of *both* exercises.

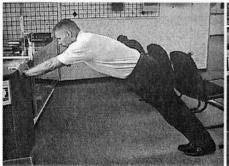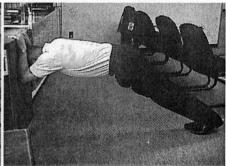

<u>Forearms</u> are next. Using your suitcase, do forearm curls for 10 reps.

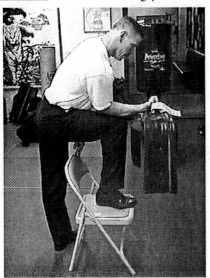 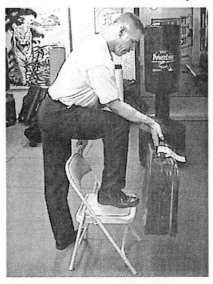

Next, put your hands together in a prayer position and push down to stretch. Repeat for three sets. Using a set of hand squeezers (you can buy them at just about any sports department), squeeze 30 times with each hand. A tennis ball will also work. Repeat for three sets.

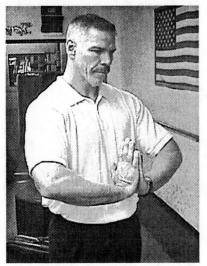 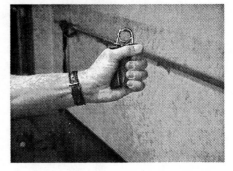

You're going to love this one. For the <u>shoulders,</u> we are going to do an exercise that has six movements rolled into one. Start with a light weight, (and I mean light: four to six pounds). What can you use for weight? You can use phone books in your hotel room or your computer case and your empty suitcase.

- Start with lateral raises to the front for 10,
- then outward to the side for 10,
- then do 10 elbow raises,
- then do 10 surges,
- then do 10 military presses, and
- then do 10 bent-over flies, (whew). Do three sets. (I told you that was a good one!)

We are now going to finish off with the same <u>ab</u> work you did on the first day of this level. Day three is the day you take off. This program runs for one week.

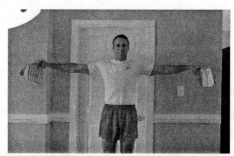

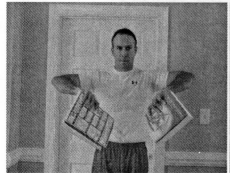

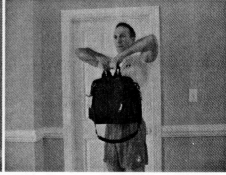

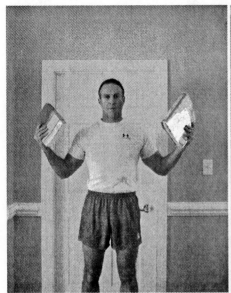
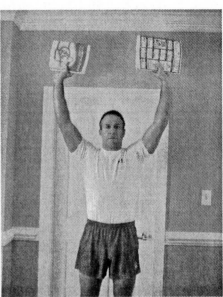
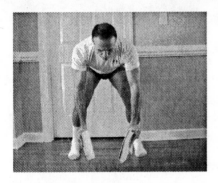
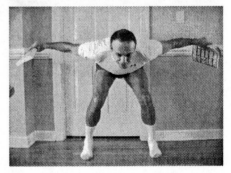

In week three of this level we will add reps.

<u>Chest</u>: Increase exercise from 10 to 12 reps on the push-ups to 12 to 15. Also increase the chair dips from10 reps to 12.

<u>Back</u>: Increase exercise from 10 to 12 reps on the wide base push-ups to 12 to 15. On your door pull-ups add two more reps.

<u>Legs</u>: Add 5 reps to your chair squats (increase from 10 reps to 15 reps). On the lunges go from 10 to 15.

<u>Arms</u>: Increase your biceps and triceps super-sets from 10 to 12.

<u>Forearms</u>: Add two curls (to 12) and try for 50 reps on the hand squeezers.

<u>Shoulders</u>: Increase weight from four to six pounds, to six to eight pounds.

<u>Abs</u>: Do 20 crunches, 20/20 knee presses, 20 elbow-to-knee presses on both sides, and 20 elbow crunches (Elbow crunches, incidentally, are done by putting your elbows by your sides with your fists pointing straight up and pushing yourself up as high as you can and then coming back down).

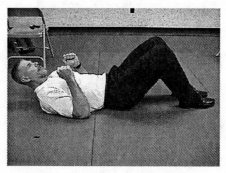

Now we've completed six weeks and should be ready for the advanced program.

Advanced Program

On this advanced program we work four days on and one off. This time we will switch, doing chest, back, and legs on one day and arms and shoulders on the next.

<u>Chest</u>: First are push-ups done with a wide base, but with fingers pointed straight ahead. Do four sets of 20 reps. Next, do peck chair dips (see pictures on page 86): put two chairs back-to-back and shoulder-width apart. Place a pillow in the middle, and use hand towels to cushion your

grip. With your chin tucked down to your chest, lower yourself down to the pillow and raise yourself up. Do four sets of 12 reps.

<u>Back</u>: Do push-ups with an extra wide base, fingers pointed out. Do four sets of 20 reps. For door pull-ups, use a towel on the top of the door, and make sure that the door will support your weight. Pull yourself up as high as you can and lower yourself slowly. Do as many as you can for four sets.

<u>Legs</u>: Standing just in front of a chair with your feet shoulder-width apart and your toes facing slightly out, squat down until your bottom barely touches the chair. Hold your hands and arms out in front of you for balance. Do one set of 50. For lunges, step forward with your right leg until your left knee almost touches the floor, then step back to the original position and back out again. Do this 20 times, then repeat with your other leg for one set.

Next, get on your hands and knees, keeping your stomach tight, and kick back with your heel, bringing your leg back to the starting position and out again. Do this 20 times on each leg.

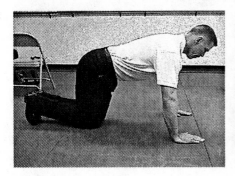 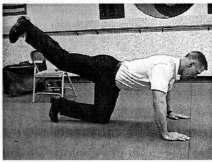

Then *without resting,* do 20 side raises with each leg. Go right into straight leg raises to the back. Do 20 with each leg.

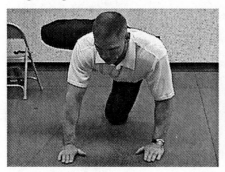 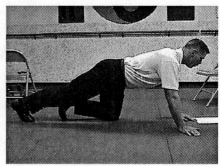

Last is the sidekick: bring your knee to your triceps and kick out at a 45-degree angle 20 times with each leg. That, my friends, will give you an "RHB"—a round, hard bottom.

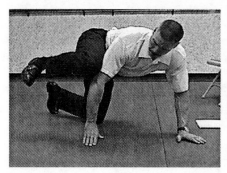 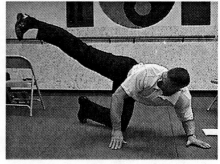

End the day with <u>abs</u>. Start with crunches: while lying on the floor, put your hands on your temples and crunch up until your shoulders and upper back are off the floor. Do 20 reps, then move right into knee presses at 20/20. Grab your shin and try to bring your knee as close to your chin as you can while holding your other foot off the ground *only* 6 inches. Count "one, two, three, *one,*" then switch legs and count "one, two, three, *two,*" and so on until you get to 20. Then do the same thing without using your hands to pull you up for another 20. Cross your left foot over your right knee, and put your right hand on your temple; then bring your right elbow to your left knee. Do this 20 times and repeat on the other side.

Now for two-second crunches: with your knees bent, crunch upward with your hands reaching for the ceiling and hold for two counts ("one-one thousand, two-one thousand, *one...*"), then release and move back down.

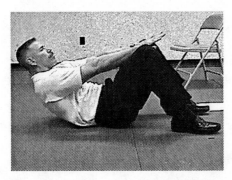

Crunch up again, but this time reach through your knees toward the wall and count "one-one thousand, two-one thousand, *three...*". Repeat these two moves for 20 reps. Next, put your elbows on the floor next to your ribs. With your closed fists pointing straight up, crunch up by pushing down on your elbows and lifting yourself up as high as you can. Do one set. Then we're done for today...yea!

Arms and Shoulders Day:

<u>Biceps and triceps</u>: We will super-set these exercises. (Remember that super-setting means doing biceps and triceps together without rest in between muscle groups.) Start with suitcase curls. Fill your suitcase with phone books, shoes or whatever you can find. Face a wall, stand back two or three feet, put your hand on the wall, and lean forward. Curl the suitcase seven times, moving only halfway up in your full range of motion. Then curl it up seven more times, only in the top range of motion. Then curl seven last times in a full range of motion. Repeat on the other arm. These are affectionately called "7-ups."

After one set of these, go directly on to triceps without a break. For the triceps, we will do what's called "counter dips." Put your hands together on a counter edge and step back with your feet together. Dip down until you go beneath the counter or until your elbows touch the wall. Then push yourself back up. Do 10 to 12 reps; do four sets of 7-ups and counter dips.

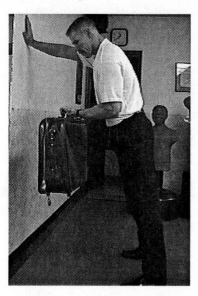
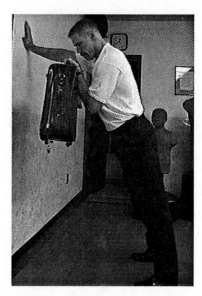

Forearms: Sit down on a chair. Using your suitcase, drape your forearm over your thigh and do 4 sets of forearm curls for 10 reps each. For the next exercise, we'll be using a piece of equipment that you can make or buy and bring with you. Get yourself a piece of wooden dowel about one foot long. Drill a hole in it that will accommodate a cord one-quarter inch or smaller in diameter. Take a piece of cord that will reach from your shoulders to the ground and thread it through the hole in the dowel. Tie a knot in it and there you have it: a "wrist roll." Attach it to your gallon jug of water and extend your arms out at shoulder height. Then roll the jug away from you until it hits the tip, then roll it back down. Do two reps for four sets. (This exercise is great for your forearms). Ok…it might be a little difficult for all you busy people to get a dowel or find time for to go to the hardware store…bottom line find things to substitute as exercise equipment. Be creative.

<u>Shoulders</u>: You can start with the six-step shoulder exercise that we covered in the intermediate program, or you can make a heavy suitcase and start with surges. Lift your suitcase up to your chin and back down; do 20 reps for four sets. Now take your suitcase and do military-style presses by lifting it over your head and down to your chest; do 15 reps for four sets. And last, for the shoulders, do incline push-ups. Place your hands shoulder-width apart with your feet close in, so your bottom is raised up. Bring your head down to touch the ground; do 10 reps for four sets.

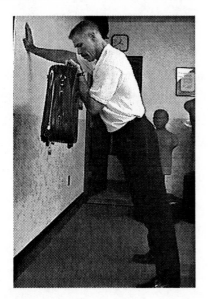 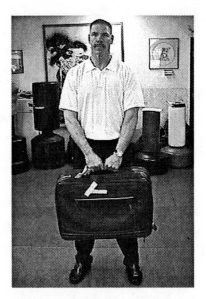

Finish off with the ab workout you did on the first day, or mix them up. Repeat the program for four days in a row, then take a day off and start it all over again.

Lastly, I give you my word: if you do this program, you will get results. Now for my last pointer: here are some ways to intensify your workouts when you're ready for a higher level of difficulty: 1) add more reps; 2) add more weight; 3) change the tempo of your workout (e.g., do them very quickly or very slowly); 4) mix routines up. Try working the all-pushing muscles one day and the all-pulling the next; or try exercising *some* pushing and *some* pulling on the same day. Whatever you do, have fun and be healthy!

When in Doubt, Talk to Your Doctor

Most businesspeople tend to be on the impatient side. We all want results and we want them now. Just as business plans, product development, and strategic objectives take time, so does your fitness and health program. Be patient. And, before you start, consult your doctor and be aware of your current condition. For any self-regulated exercise program, be aware of the following risk factors and/or medical conditions: diagnosed high blood pressure, arthritis, high cholesterol, cigarette smoking, diabetes mellitus, sedentary lifestyle, pregnancy/nursing, heart condition, and/or orthopedic problems. If you fall into any of these categories, consult your physician prior to beginning an exercise program.

Stop exercising and obtain medical advice if you observe any of the following danger signs:

- unusual fatigue
- nausea
- dizziness
- tightness in chest or any pain from the jaw to the waist
- lightheadedness
- loss of muscle control
- severe breathlessness
- blurring vision

Cooling Down

Cooling down is the best way to reduce next-day soreness. However, stretching is *only part of the cooling down process*. After you have completed your workout, the best way to reduce muscle fatigue and soreness (caused by the production of lactic acid from your maximal or near-maximal muscle exertion) is to perform a light *warm-down*. This warm-down is similar to the second half of your warm-up (but in the reverse order). The warm-down consists of the following phases:

1. sport-specific activity,

2. dynamic stretching, and

3. static stretching.

Ideally, you should start your warm-down with about 10 to 20 minutes of sport-specific activity (perhaps only a little more intense than in your warm-up). In reality, however, you may not always have 10 to 20 minutes to spare at the end of your workout. In this case, you should attempt to perform at least five minutes of sport-specific activity. The sport-specific activity should immediately be followed by stretching: first, perform some light dynamic stretches until your heart rate slows down to its normal rate, then perform some static stretches. Sport-specific activity, followed by stretching, can reduce cramping, tightening, and soreness in fatigued muscles, and will make you feel better after workouts.

When You're Cooped Up: Exercising in a Confined Space

Exercises While Sitting in a Plane or Automobile

Have you ever been trapped in an airplane in a middle row seat sitting on the runway for two hours? Maybe you have experienced traffic jams where your car is motionless for hours. In situation like these, sitting in one spot can make you feel terrible. Even when sitting or standing for prolonged periods of time, you can perform a few exercises that help increase blood circulation and maintain flexibility. Here are a few exercises that can help:

Neck and Upper Back Exercises

Maintain good posture and alignment by sitting tall, with your shoulders back but relaxed, your pelvis in neutral alignment, and your head positioned as if someone were pulling your hair straight up. Breathe normally. Repeat each of the following repetitions slowly and with control.

1. While sitting or standing, slowly tilt your head towards your right shoulder, leading with the right ear. The action is as if you were placing your right ear close to your right shoulder. Hold this position for three to five seconds, then slowly tilt your head toward your left shoulder and hold. Repeat a few times to both sides.

2. Lift your shoulders to your ears (shoulder shrug), then lower to your starting position. Do this four or five times.

3. Turn your head slowly to the right side, looking over right shoulder. Turn your head and neck as far as it feels comfortable. Hold for three to five seconds, then slowly turn your head to left side, looking as far over left shoulder as possible. Repeat a few times to each side, moving slowly and with control.

4. Round your shoulders forward, then press them back, squeezing your shoulder blades together. Repeat, moving slowly and with control. Exhale when you round your shoulders forward and inhale when you press your shoulders back, lifting the chest, and sitting tall at the same time. Repeat at a slow to moderate pace five times. Then gently rotate your shoulders front, up, back, and down; repeat five times.

5. Reach both arms to the front of your body, interlacing your fingers. With your arms reaching to the front, relax your shoulders, let your head lower naturally downward as your eyes focus between your arms. Relax into this upper-back stretch and maintain steady rhythmic breathing.

Buttock Exercises

1. Sitting or standing tall, contract your buttocks slowly to a four-count contraction. Then slowly release on four counts. Repeat several times.

2. When sitting, roll and transfer weight to your right hip and buttock as you lift the left hip off the seat. Roll to your left hip, transferring your weight as you lift your right hip off the seat. Perform this motion slowly and with control in an easy rolling side-to-side fashion. Do not perform this exercise if you have a back injury.

Lower Body Exercises

1. While sitting or standing tall, march in place for 30 counts. Let your arms swing freely at your sides. Don't worry if someone stares at you. Remember: you're trying to feel better—not trying impress someone you don't know.

2. While sitting, lift your right foot. Slowly point and then flex your right foot to stretch the shin and calf. Repeat on your left foot. Slowly rotate your right ankle in a clockwise direction, then slowly reverse direction. Repeat on the left ankle. This exercise will help to relieve stiffness in your joints.

3. Bring your right knee into your chest, stretching the buttock and lower back. Hold. Release, then repeat the stretch by bringing your left knee to your chest.

Hand and Wrist Exercises

1. Open and close your hands, stretching fingers as far as they can comfortably open, then close, forming a fist. This exercise is great in helping to reduce the fluid retention in your hands. Do this exercise until you feel a slight tingling or burning sensation. Relax and then repeat for two to three sets.
2. Rotate your wrists, circling inward, then outward.

The Run: Short but Effective Runs for the Road Warrior

One of the best feelings while traveling is getting out of an airplane after a three-hour flight. If your schedule allows it, go to the hotel and change into your workout uniform. Complete a short warm-up and stretch, then hit the road running. Not enough time? Here is a great quick work out.

The Sprint

Equipment: running shoes, shorts, and a football field or park

1. After a good warm-up, run a 100-yard dash at one-half your sprint speed.
2. At the end of 100 yards, do an easy jog back to the starting point. Then sprint 100 yards at three-quarters your full speed.
3. Now do 100 yards at full speed, jogging back to the starting point for six repetitions. This is a high intensity work out. If you can get all your repetitions in without throwing up, you are in great shape. If you feel a little sick, slow down a bit and/or reduce the number of reps.

The Shuttle Run

This is a very good running workout that burns loads of calories while improving your agility as well. Run back and forth between two markers. Run in a straight line as fast as you can. When you reach the marker opposite from where you started, bend down to touch the ground, and with a burst, run back to the other end of the ground where you began. Repeat this action for at least five laps, running back and forth. Football and basketball players and other athletes use shuttle runs to improve their agility and strength. Shuttle runs will do wonders for your softball game when you're trying to outrun that shortstop. Word of caution to you former Jocks with bad knees…do this only if it does not hurt. There is no "good" pain in the shuttle run.

If you have time to get in a good day's run, the following runs are focused on burning calories.

Interval Hi-Lo Runs

Run at 75 to 90 percent of your maximum for one mile, then alternate it with jogging at 70 percent of your maximum speed to recover for five minutes (or half a mile—whichever comes first). Keep alternating the running and jogging for the length of your work out. (I recommend at least a good 30 minutes.) This stress-recovery workout will help you: build a higher tolerance for running, run further than you would have within the same amount of time, and get your metabolism to burn more calories because it won't plateau. You'll not only burn calories, but your body will remain at a higher metabolic rate hours after you have finished your workout.

If You Have the Time: The Long Run

Run at a slow pace for 45 minutes to an hour. Running at a slow pace for 45 minutes or more will maximize total fat burning. If you're not in running shape, don't just start with a one-hour run. Build yourself up.

Walk at first. Start your running program with a pace that you can do comfortably. Every week, run for five minutes longer than the week before until you reach 45 to 60 minutes.

Morning Runs

When you wake up, before you eat anything, go out for a quick 30-minute run. When you exercise first thing, your body will use fat for energy because it used your stored carbohydrates while you were sleeping. Initially, exercising in the morning may make you feel like sampling everything on the buffet line, but you will burn more calories because your body will feel like it needs more energy.

Example Workout

The Warm-up

1. Start off with walking around the track for one lap.
2. Jog one lap around the track at 60 to 70 percent of your maximum speed.
3. Do some light skipping for three minutes.
4. March in place for 30 seconds.
5. Lightly stretch your chest, triceps, quadriceps, hamstrings, and calves. (This should take about a minute or so; hold each stretch for eight seconds.)

The Workout

1. Lunges (12 repetitions per leg)
2. Jumping jacks (12 repetitions)
3. Hamstring curls (12 reps per leg)
4. Calf raises (12 reps per leg)

5. Run one lap around the track at 85 percent of your maximum speed.

6. Push-ups (15 on feet, 10 on knees)

7. Back stabilizer exercise (12 reps for each side)

8. Fly-ups (12 reps)

9. Ab crunches with a twist (12 reps for each side)

10. Run one lap around the track.

11. Do triceps dips with one leg up (12 reps per leg)

12. Bicep curls (12 reps each arm)

13. Squats without weights (12 reps)

14. Jump rope for 30 seconds

The Cool Down

1. Walk one lap around the track.

2. Take a pulse check—it should be around 80 percent of its maximum rate.

3. Stretch, starting from the bottom to the top. Hold each stretch for a good 10 to 15 seconds; if the muscle feels sore, repeat the stretch and hold it for another 10 to 15 seconds. Stretch:

    *   calves
    *   hamstrings
    *   hip flexors
    *   quadriceps
    *   chest
    *   triceps
    *   cat stretch – Yes…stretch just like your cat or dog. I know it looks silly, so do it when no one is looking.

- full arm stretch
- neck rolls, neck stretch

Shake out any kinks and drink a glass of liquid to replenish the fluid lost during the exercise.

A Word of Caution About Heat, Exercise, And Hydration

(http://www.angelfire.com/me/loulou77/heatinjuries.html)

When traveling to the sun belt, the tropics, or a hot-humid place, be cautious about overdoing it. Pushing your body too hard in the heat can cause major health problems. Before you exercise in the heat, you should evaluate the potential heat/stress danger that results from the combination of temperature and humidity. If it's hot and humid outside, your safest bet is to go swimming or seek the controlled environment of an air-conditioned exercise facility.

Hydration

The body's need for water is second in importance only to its need for oxygen. Water accounts for approximately 55 to 60 percent of our adult body weight. As we exercise and use our muscles, we generate internal heat that's dissipated by sweating. Through the evaporation of sweat, we can keep cool throughout a workout. Furthermore, sweating has a cleansing effect that rids the body of impurities. So sweating without re-hydrating your body can cause headaches, muscle cramps, light-headedness, fatigue, lethargy, and persistent elevated body temperature. Make certain you're consuming enough fluids to adequately hydrate your body—it is recommended that you drink 8 to 10 glasses of fluids daily (8 ounces per glass). Ingest fluids before, during, and after exercise and don't rely on your thirst mechanism to tell you how much fluid you need. Also, avoid drinks that contain caffeine (e.g., coffee, soft drinks, and tea) or alcohol (e.g., beer, wine, etc.); they can increase both urine production and fluid loss.

Heat Injury Prevention

The following are actions that you can take to help prevent dehydration during exercise:

1. The best way to prevent dehydration is to hydrate your body before working out. Consume 8 to 10 ounces of water 10 to 20 minutes before beginning a light workout.

2. Follow the warm-up procedures outlined in this book. The warm-up phase of exercise gradually increases your body temperature, allowing the body's sweat mechanism to help cool you.

3. When exercising for an hour or more, take breaks to consume additional water. Recommended intake is 3 ounces every 20 minutes.

4. All you former high school athletes, this one is for you: *avoid salt tablets.* Sweat is composed primarily of water lost from tissues. Given that you lose more water than sodium and chloride, this means that the body is under pressure to correct the imbalance. For this reason, additional salt or salt tablets are undesirable prior to or after strenuous exercise. Use water to prevent heat injury or thermal stress.

5. Wear clothing that allows for evaporation and ventilation. Appropriate dress during exercise is another important consideration in the prevention of heat stress. This involves dressing in light, loose-fitting clothing during hot weather exercise, especially on humid days when your body's sweating mechanism is less efficient.

6. On very hot days, stay indoors or in the shade. Exercising in full sun increases the risk of heat injury. Covering your head guards against the sun's radiant energy and will help protect you from dehydration as well as sunburn.

7. If you become overheated, moisten your skin by sponging or spraying with water to assist in the cooling process. Fans may aid evaporation.

Such cooling measures provide a form of external sweating, which helps to dissipate heat without using internal fluid reserves for evaporation.

Common Exercise Misconceptions

There are numerous opinions regarding the components of the ideal exercise program. Unfortunately, much of the information supporting these opinions is either completely false or born of half-truths leading to common misperceptions. Many movie stars and renowned "beautiful people" on television commercials are simply pushing products. Not all of them are bad, but I bet you dollars to donuts that Suzanne Summers is doing more then just the Thigh Buster to maintain her figure. In the same way that you scrutinize a new product before you buy, examine the areas of an exercise program that will work for you. That means that you shouldn't spend your time doing the eight-minute abdominal workout when you really need overall fitness to reduce your love handles.

Over the years, I've collected some common misconceptions on fitness. Maybe you've heard the same statements from your colleagues or from the person seating next to you on the airplane.

Misconception 1:

"I weigh about the same as I did in high school, so I'm still in pretty good shape."

Reality:

Chances are that the weight, once in the chest and arms, is now around the mid-section. Lack of exercise diminishes our muscle tissue and increases our body fat. This sad fact of the sedentary lifestyle has a direct negative effect on our level of fitness, even if the bathroom scale does not reflect the change.

Misconception 2:

"If I want to lose weight, I should just exercise aerobically and not lift weights."

Reality:

Losing weight is primarily a factor of burning calories and/or reduction in caloric intake. Lean muscle uses fat as a fuel when conducting aerobic exercise. Muscle weighs more than fat. A combination of resistance exercises and aerobic exercise is the correct approach to total fitness. To condition muscle tissue, perform the Anderson exercise routine. This will help the body to burn fat more efficiently when exercising.

Misconception 3:

"I know I got a good workout when I am really sore for days afterward."

Reality:

Your hard-core trainer may be saying to you, "No pain, No gain." It is true that we cause microscopic tears to our muscles when we train with heavy weights. However, you should not be sore after every workout. Instead, plan to gradually increase the amount of weight or difficulty only 5 to 10 percent every six workouts.

Misconception 4:

"I know I've had a good workout if I sweat a lot."

Reality:

I sweat a lot when I eat spicy food. Some people sweat when they have to speak in public. Some people sweat when the temperature is above 70 degrees Fahrenheit. Do not gauge your workout on how much you sweat. Sweating is the body's way of cooling itself off and varies dramatically among individuals.

Misconception 5:

"When I feel tightness, cramping, or slight pain during exercise, I just keep trying to stretch the muscle out."

Reality:

This is a difficult one for the tough women and men of the world. Admittedly some muscle cramps can be stretched out successfully in order to resume exercise. However, spasms or contractions of muscle fiber can be caused by a variety of conditions from electrolyte imbalance to injury. Cramping is actually the body's own protective mechanism, signaling you to stop in order to limit further damage. The best rule of thumb is this: If the muscle spasm cannot be relieved by one or two simple stretches, then you may be experiencing a prelude to an injury. Stop the activity, apply ice, elevate, and compress the injured body part. If it continues to hurt, consult your physician.

Misconception 6:

"Lifting weights will put too much stress on my joints."

Reality:

You always hear this one from folks with "bad" backs or "bad" knees. Actually the opposite is true. Joints become healthier with resistance training. Obviously, overloading a joint can lead to an injury. Injuries happen when the joint is overloaded and your body is not warmed and stretched correctly or has already been injured previously. However, if you do the correct form of resistance training, with a full range of motion and without overloading, you will strengthen your joints as well as your connective tissues (ligaments and tendons).

Misconception 7:

"As a woman, I don't want to lift weights because I don't want big bulky muscles."

Reality:

Don't worry, it won't happen. Unless women are into serious body-building and weightlifting they will not get bulky muscles. Women do not produce enough of the hormone testosterone for hypertrophy to occur. However, women can expect to achieve attractive toning and def-inition from resistance training.

Misconception 8:

"If I stop weight training, the muscles I've developed will turn into fat."

Reality:

I hear this one all the time. **Muscles cannot turn into fat**. One cannot become the other. However, stopping your resistance-training program may allow the developed muscle tissue to atrophy (shrink). If you are eating the same amount of calories but using fewer calories, new fat deposits will develop. The decreased muscle tone, combined with new fat deposits caused by a lack of exercise, tend to give the appearance of muscle that has turned to fat.

Misconception 9:

"I'm really working on my flexibility, so I don't need to do the aerobic or weight training thing."

Reality:

Flexibility is only part of your well-being; flexibility by itself will not keep you healthy.

Chapter Eight

Returning to the Home Front: Putting It All Together

It's been a tough trip. You've survived intense meetings, long flights, and stressful traveling companions. You're looking forward to getting home. Yet now you realize that your friends and family have survived without you; they have continued going to school or work and lived their lives in your absence. At work, decisions have been made and customers have been taken care of, all without you. It is hard for you to imagine, but the world didn't stop while you were away. Oftentimes, people underestimate the issues surrounding your readjustment to your family, social, and professional life. Returning home, even from a brief trip, can sometimes be more traumatic than leaving.

Family and Friends

During your trip, you can help ease your transition home by keeping in close communication: call home or use e-mail to stay in touch. If you have little ones, it helps for them to know that Mommy or Daddy cares, even while they're away. Let your family know what time of the day you are returning. Find out what their schedule is and adjust your return celebration accordingly (even if you've been gone for less then a week). If the children are at school, take your spouse or friend to lunch. If you usually arrive home tired from your trip, take a quick power nap or have some quiet time with someone special. The trick is this: plan your return before you leave. Set up a block of time that you can dedicate to the special people in your life.

Work

Returning from your trip on a Friday or Saturday (if you can) tends to be much less stressful than returning on a Sunday. Having an extra day to get home, unpack, and relax before returning to the office can be invaluable. While traveling, remember that communication is key; stay in touch with your work associates and stay on top of major projects and schedules. Otherwise you may have to play catch up and immediately start using your stress-reduction techniques. Everyone has routines for returning; here's one that works well for me:

❑ Unpack your briefcase or travel bag immediately.

❑ Sort through your mail, typically creating three piles: 1) Urgent 2) Important 3) Junk. Then address the urgent mail and trash your junk mail. Though it may seem simple, organizing your mail helps to bring closure and a sense of accomplishment.

❑ Sort through your e-mail and voice mail in the same fashion. There should be significantly less e-mail and voice mail if you've been clearing your messages every day while traveling.

❑ Change your voice-mail message to reflect your return.

❑ Talk to your boss and your direct reports to ensure there isn't a "hot" issue that needs to be addressed immediately.

The information covered in this book is tried and tested. It works. If you follow the guidelines of this book, we guarantee that you will achieve your traveling health and fitness goals. Even more importantly, the changes you make to your daily routine will have a positive effect on every aspect of your life. You owe it to yourself, your family, your employer, and your career to take care of yourself. Think about it: how effective and efficient can you be if you don't take care of yourself? One of my former co-workers recently passed away. The coroner declared a heart attack as the cause, due to an unhealthy lifestyle. He was stressed, overweight, and unable to sleep; all in all he was a physical train wreck. Face it: these days, nobody is expecting you to work until you drop. The scrooges of the world were pushed out of the corporate corner office in the re-engineering and downsizing of the early 1990s. *Results* are what matter in the business world, and you won't get results if you're dead or deathly ill.

Your health and well-being are priceless. It's nearly impossible to enjoy the financial rewards of success when your body is worn-out or broken. These days, for better or worse, most businesspeople must travel to be successful. While the Internet, fax, and cell phones have greatly *increased* our productivity, the need to build relationships and interface directly with our customers and employers in this global village may increase our need to travel. So take the holistic approach to maintaining your health. If you have been able to stay fit on the road, employ those same techniques to keep you healthy at home. Visualize your goals, set your program, and make it happen!

Appendix

Discussion on Heart Rate

Your heart rate is the number of times your heart beats, or contracts, every minute. Measuring your recovery rate—the rate at which your heart rate decreases to normal after a workout—is a way to evaluate your fitness level after exercise. For example, you exercise for half an hour at 155 beats per minute. Two minutes after you stop exercising, your heart rate decreases to 95. So, 95 beats per minute is your recovery heart rate. Set a two-minute time frame and see how many beats you recover within those two minutes. Then compare this recovery rate with future exercise sessions.

Your resting heart rate indicates your basic fitness level. Your resting heart rate (Resting HR) is the number of heartbeats occurring in one minute when you are at rest. The more fit you are, the less effort and fewer beats per minute it takes your heart to pump blood while your body is at rest. Your maximum heart rate (Max HR) is the highest number of times your heart can contract in one minute. Max HR is the most useful tool for determining training intensities, because it can be individually measured or predicted.

How do you determine your maximum heart rate?

You can have it measured at a clinic. Typically your Max HR test will be done on a treadmill. A mathematical formula allows you to predict your Max HR with some accuracy; it's called the "age-adjusted formula." The age-adjusted Max HR formula can come in very handy when you're not prepared to pay for the physician-supervised stress test.

WOMEN: 226 - your age = age-adjusted Max HR
MEN: 220 - your age = age-adjusted Max HR

So, for example: if you are a 30-year-old woman, your age-adjusted maximum heart rate is 226 - 30 years = 196 bpm (beats per minute). It should be noted that these formulas apply only to adults. The generally accepted margin of error in the age-predicted formula is plus or minus 10 to 15 beats per minute, which is due both to different inherited characteristics and exercise training. The formula will give you an estimate to work from, but if you want to exercise or train at your most effective levels, your Max HR should be measured professionally.

Your Target Zone

Using your **target zone** means letting the range of your heart rate guide your workout. By this I mean keeping your intensity level between an upper and lower heart-rate limit. Various target zones that correspond with your specific exercise goals are suggested below for you to follow.

Train Effectively—Use the Zones

If you're a beginner whose goals are improving overall fitness, losing weight, or reducing stress, make sure you exercise in the **healthy heart** zone (50 to 60 percent of your maximum heart rate). If you already exercise regularly, but are aiming to lose body fat, exercise in the **weight management** zone (60 to 70 percent of your maximum heart rate). Build yourself up to a workout of an hour of continuous exercise. If your goal is to improve your aerobic capacity or athletic performance, exercise in the **aerobic** zone (70 to 80 percent of your maximum heart rate).

Competitive athletes may need to add interval training sessions during the week in the **anaerobic threshold heart rate** zone, which is 80 to 90 percent of maximum. This high-intensity exercise helps train muscles to handle lactic acid. Remember, though, to train sparingly at these upper limits. Exercising regularly at a very high heart rate does not produce additional aerobic benefits, and it increases the possibility of an athletic injury. Interval training and anaerobic threshold workouts require a high degree of fitness and are not necessary for general fitness training.

Cardiovascular endurance, or aerobic fitness, is the ability to exercise continuously for extended periods without tiring, an important component of many sporting activities.

A person's aerobic fitness level is dependent upon the amount of oxygen that can be transported by the body to the working muscles, and the muscles' level of efficiency in using that oxygen. The best test for aerobic fitness is the **maximal oxygen uptake** (VO_{2max}) test. As this test can be both expensive and time consuming, many other simpler tests have been designed to predict a VO_{2max} score. The many tests for aerobic fitness can be divided into either **maximal** or **submaximal** tests. Stressing the body by exercising to exhaustion (as in the maximal tests) is sometimes not appropriate, therefore the submaximal tests, which are less demanding (and also usually less accurate), can be used.

Run Test for Set Time or Distance

- **Description/Procedure:** There are several tests that involve running for a set time (e.g. 9, 10, or 12 minutes) or a set distance (1 mile, 1.5 miles, or 1,200 meters), and recording the distance covered or time required. The time required for these tests normally ranges from 8 to 15 minutes, depending on the population being tested.

- **Modifications:** In addition to different times and distances used for this test, different exercise modes (such as swimming) can be used. See also the submaximal **walk tests** below.

- **Scoring:** Norms for males and females for the one-mile run and nine-minute run are published in the *AAHPERD Manual* (1980).

There are equations that you can use to estimate VO_{2max} from performance in these tests; for example, for the 12-minute run, VO_{2max} (in ml/kg/min) = (35.97 x miles) - 11.29.

- **Target Population:** This test can be modified for divergent populations. For adults, the test should last at least 10 minutes to ensure that energy demands are supplied by the aerobic system. Shorter runs are more suitable for children.

- **Equipment Required:** An oval or running track, marking cones, recording sheets, and a stopwatch.

- **Validity:** Cooper (1968) reported a correlation of 0.90 between VO_{2max} and the distance covered in a 12-minute walk/run. Other studies generally have a correlation of 0.65 or better for runs of greater than nine minutes (or a mile).

- **Reliability:** The reliability of the test would depend on practice and pacing strategies and motivation level. The test should be reliable if the aforementioned issues are addressed.

- **Advantages:** Large groups can be tested at once, and it is a very cheap and simple test to perform.

- **Disadvantages:** Practice and pacing is required, and performance on this test can be affected greatly by motivation.

References:

Cooper, K.H. (1968). A Means of Assessing Maximal Oxygen Uptake. Journal of the American Medical Association 203:201-204.

Two-Kilometer Walk Test

- **Description:** This test involves a brisk walking performance followed by simple measurements. It provides direct information on walking fitness (time and heart rate) and can be used to predict maximal oxygen uptake.

- **Scoring:** The results are calculated from the following: a) how long the two-kilometer walk takes, b) heart rate at the end of the walk, c) **body mass index** and, d) age. You can study norms to place your individual scores within a fitness category.

- **Equipment Required:** You'll need a stopwatch, a marked two-kilometer track or path on level ground with a firm and smooth surface, and a heart rate monitor (optional).

- **Target Population:** Adults aged 20 to 65 who are in poor fitness and would not be able to complete a run test.

- **Reliability:** This test is highly reliable, except with people with a high VO_{2max}.

- **Advantages:** There is minimal equipment and cost involved, and the test can be administered either independently or to large groups at once.

- **Disadvantages:** It can be too easy for the highly fit.

Reference:

Taken from the Eurofit for adults book: *Assessment of Health Related Fitness*, by the Council of Europe Publishing.

Body Mass Index

Body composition refers primarily to the distribution of muscle and fat in the body, and its measurement plays an important role in both sports and health. Excess body fat may lead to obesity and increases your susceptibility to many diseases. In sports, excess fat hinders performance, as it doesn't contribute to muscular force production, and, after all, it requires extra energy to move fat around.

Body composition is often represented as a two-compartment system: lean body weight and fat weight. The fat weight is expressed as a percentage of total body weight, where percent body fat = (fat weight / total body weight) x 100. The table below gives general guidelines for body fat percentage levels.

	GENERAL POPULATION		ATHLETES	
	Males	Females	Males	Females
Lean	< 12	< 17	< 7	< 12
Acceptable	12 - 21	17 - 28	7 - 15	12 - 25
Moderately Overweight	21 - 26	28 - 33		
Overweight	> 26	> 33	> 15	> 25

Many training or exercise programs are geared solely to modify your body size and composition in some way. The tests described below provide a way of measuring your current levels and determining changes over time.

- **Description/Procedure:** BMI is calculated from **body mass** (M) and **height** (H). BMI = M / (H x H), where M = body mass in kilograms and H = height in meters. The higher the score the higher the levels of body fat.

Scoring:

Underweight	<20
Healthy Range	20-25
Overweight	25-30
Obese	>30

- **Equipment Required:** You'll need scales and a stadiometer to measure weight and height.
- **Target Population:** BMI is often used to determine the level of health risk associated with obesity.
- **Advantages:** Simple calculation from standard measurements.
- **Disadvantages:** BMI can be inaccurate. For example, lean athletes who are large and muscular could score high BMI levels, which would incorrectly rate them as obese.
- **Other Comments:** There are other, more accurate measures of body composition that would be preferable if available.

Hip—Waist Ratio

- **Description/Procedure:** This is a simple calculation of the measurements of your **waist girth** divided by the **hip girth.**
- **Scoring:** The table below gives general guidelines for acceptable levels for hip to waist ratio.

	ACCEPTABLE		UNACCEPTABLE		
	Excellent	Good	Average	High	Extreme
Male	< 0.85	0.85 - 0.90	0.90 - 0.95	0.95 - 1.00	> 1.00
Female	< 0.75	0.75 - 0.80	0.80 - 0.85	0.85 - 0.90	> 0.90

- **Equipment Required:** You'll need a tape measure.

- **Target Population:** This measure is often used to determine the coronary artery disease risk associated with obesity. The target population would then be anyone in a high-risk category.

- **Advantages:** A simple measure that can be taken at home by people to monitor their own levels.

- **Other Comments:** The basis of this measure as a coronary disease risk factor follows the assumption that fat stored around the waist poses a greater risk to health than fat stored elsewhere. Average is in the "unacceptable" range as we would like you to strive for "Good". For more information on this topic, go to: http://www.worldfitness.org/exer0002.html.

0-595-26079-9

Printed in the United States
60800LVS00004B/112-180

9 780595 260799